TREATMENT OF RADIORESISTANT CANCERS

TREATMENT OF RADIORESISTANT CANCERS

Proceedings of the International Symposium on the Prospects for Treatment of Radioresistant Cancers held in Kyoto (Japan), May 21, 1979.

Editors:

M. Abe

K. Sakamoto

and

T.L. Phillips

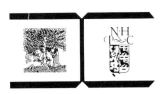

1979

ELSEVIER/NORTH-HOLLAND BIOMEDICAL PRESS

AMSTERDAM · NEW YORK · OXFORD

© 1979 Elsevier/North-Holland Biomedical Press

ISBN: 0-444-80179-0

Published by:
Elsevier/North-Holland Biomedical Press
335 Jan van Galenstraat, P.O. Box 211
Amsterdam, The Netherlands

Sole distributors for the USA and Canada:
Elsevier North Holland Inc.
52 Vanderbilt Avenue
New York, N.Y. 10017

Library of Congress Cataloging in Publication Data
International Symposium on the Prospects for
    Treatment of Radioresistant Cancers, Kyoto,
    1979.
    Treatment of radioresistant cancers.

    Bibliography: p.
    Includes index.
    1. Cancer--Radiotherapy--Congresses.
2. Radiation-sensitizing agents--Congresses.
3. Thermotherapy--Congresses. I. Abe,
Mitsuyuki, 1932-   II. Sakamoto, Kiyohiko,
1933-   III. Phillips, Theodore L.
IV. Title. [DNLM: 1. Radioimmunoassay--
Congresses. 2. Catecholamines--Analysis--
Congresses. 3. Prostaglandins--Analysis--
Congresses. 4. Cardiovascular agents--Agents--
Analysis--Congresses. 5. Hypertension--
Congresses. 5. Endorphins--Analysis--
Congresses. W3 SY1056 v. 3 1979 / QV150 I590r
1979]
RC271.R3I55 1979   616.9'94'07   79-22400
ISBN 0-444-80179-0

Printed in The Netherlands

PREFACE

With the advent of megavoltage sources, significant improvements in the cure rate of malignant disease have been achieved in radiotherapy. However, there are two limiting factors in current radiotherapy which have remained unresolved. One is that there exists highly radioresistant tumors such as osteosarcoma or hypoxic tumor cells which can hardly be eliminated by so called low LET radiation. The other is that if the tumor located near the radio-sensitive critical structures, cancerocidal doses cannot be delivered. We must also admit that local failure is unfortunately still common even with the aid of megavoltage beams.

In this sense, we must say that radiotherapy has come to a turning point. The time has come for us to seek other radiation sources beyond photons or find biological methods to overcome these problems.

The purpose of this symposium is to explore ways to approach the resolution of these problems by physical and biological means. In the physical approach to these problems, enthusiasm has arisen for the study of high LET particles in clinical radiotherapy based on potential physical and biological advantages over the use of photons and electrons. The trial use of high LET radiations such as neutrons, heavy ions, pions as an alternative or additive to photon radiotherapy is actively underway in a number of centers. The results reported from these centers are most attractive. In the biological approach, chemical agents have been examined which will overcome the radioresistant hypoxic cells. We can, now, accept that chemicals exist which have the advantage of specifically sensitizing hypoxic tumor cells, while not affecting normal tissues. We also know that the combination of hyperthermia and radiation has the potential to become a powerful tool in the treatment of cancers.

It is for this reason, I think, that this symposium may be said to come at a most appropriate time. It is the purpose of this volume to review the current status of hyperthermia, hypoxic cell sensitizers and high LET radiations in radiotherapy and to suggest new approaches to the treatment of radioresistant cancers.

Mitsuyuki Abe
Department of Radiology
Kyoto University

CONTENTS

FUNDAMENTAL AND CLINICAL APPROACHES TO RADIORESISTANT CANCERS

HYPOXIC CELL SENSITIZERS

© 1979, Elsevier/North-Holland Biomedical Press
Treatment of Radioresistant Cancers
M. Abe, K. Sakamoto and T.L. Phillips eds.

RADIATION SENSITIZERS FOR HYPOXIC CELLS: PROBLEMS AND PROSPECTS

G.E. ADAMS

Physics Division, Institute of Cancer Research, Clifton Avenue,
Sutton, Surrey (England).

INTRODUCTION

Despite the advanced treatment methods now available in radiotherapy, failure of local tumour control is a significant problem - in some sites particularly so. Although there are several reasons for this, a major cause of local failure is the problem of hypoxic cell radiation resistance. Hypoxic cells occur in a high proportion of human tumours. They arise as a result of tumour growth outstripping its blood supply and occur usually in, and around, areas of tumour necrosis[1].

Hypoxic cells are dangerous because of their relative radiation-resistance. These cells are in a resting state and would eventually die of oxygen starvation. However, subsequent to, or during, radiation treatment, tumour regression occurs due to the removal of oxic cells sterilized by the radiation. This permits some of the hypoxic cells to be re-oxygenated. They enter cycle, divide and provide a focus for the regrowth of the tumour.

Approaches to the hypoxic cell problem include treatment in hyperbaric oxygen chambers, unconventional fractionation regimes aimed at optimizing re-oxygenation processes during treatment, radiotherapy with high energy neutrons and finally radiosensitiz-drugs. Chemical agents which specifically increase the radiation sensitivity of hypoxic cells in tumours without increasing radiation damage to well-oxygenated normal tissue cells should be the preferred method of overcoming the hypoxic cell resistance. They would be cheap, and if free of complications, could be used routinely in radiotherapy without the need to invest in expensive hardware or treatment machines.

DEVELOPMENT OF HYPOXIC CELL SENSITIZERS

Many chemical compounds exist that are able to sensitize hypoxic mammalian cells to radiation although not all of these display sensitizing activity in vivo. The largest class of hypoxic cell sensitizers is the "Electron-affinic" group, so called because their relative efficiencies are a direct function of their electron affinities or reduction potentials.

The electron affinity proposal[2] led to the examination of different types of chemical structures for evidence of radiation-sensitizing properties. Compounds shown to be active in irradiated hypoxic cultures of bacterial of mammalian cells included various conjugate diketones and diesters, quinones, aromatic ketones and numerous nitroaromatic or heterocyclic compounds. Some of the structures of the early compounds are shown in Figure 1.

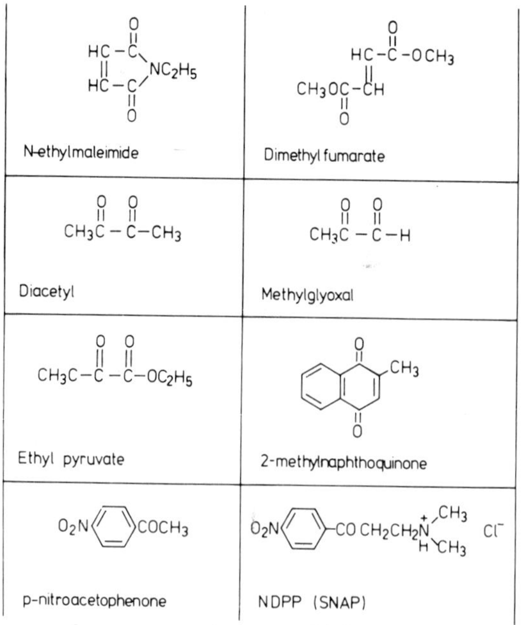

N-ethylmaleimide	Dimethyl fumarate
Diacetyl	Methylglyoxal
Ethyl pyruvate	2-methylnaphthoquinone
p-nitroacetophenone	NDPP (SNAP)

Fig. 1. Structures of some early sensitizers.

Bacterial systems were first used for assessing sensitization and many active compounds were found[3]. However, in general, little activity was found in mammalian cell systems in vitro. In 1971 the compound p.nitroacetophenone was found to be a potent sensitizer for hypoxic Chinese hamster cells irradiated in vitro[4,5]. This compound does not sensitize aerobic cells nor does the enhancement ratio for hypoxic cells vary very much with the position of the cell in the mitotic cycle. Evidence for sensitization by other nitrocompounds, the nitrofurans, soon followed[6]. This was interesting since several such compounds were in use clinically as antibiotics. However, sensitization in vivo is usually poor with these compounds since the large concentrations required for significant sensitization are often too toxic.

Although several hundred compounds of diverse chemical structure have demonstrated considerable sensitization of hypoxic cells in vitro, relatively few show pronounced activity in solid tumours in experimental animals. This is due mainly to the difficulties in penetration into the poorly-vascularized regions of tumours where hypoxic cells occur. Clearly, for a sensitizer to be effective in vivo, it must be sufficiently metabolically stable to enable it to diffuse intracellularly to the hypoxic cells which are situated probably about 150-100 microns distant from the nearest capillary.

METRONIDAZOLE AND MISONIDAZOLE

A considerable step forward occurred in 1973 with the discovery of the sensitizing action of metronidazole (Flagyl) in hypoxic bacterial and mammalian cells in culture[6,7]. Evidence soon followed of sensitization in various solid tumour systems, although the enhancement ratios observed were not large and large drug doses were generally required (for a review see references 8 and 9). Nevertheless, these results were important since they demonstrated the feasibility of the approach. Although metronidazole is relatively inefficient on a concentration basis, its half-life <u>in vivo</u> is fairly long thus apparently enabling the drug to diffuse into poorly-vascularized regions of tumours. Further encouragement followed with evidence from Urtasun and colleagues of apparent radiation sensitization of human gliomas by metronidazole[10].

The results with metronidazole led to the search for more active compounds in the nitroimidazole series. Electron affinity considerations indicated that the substituted 2-nitro-imidazoles would be better sensitizers. This was based on the expectation that a nitro group substituted in the 2-position of the imidazole ring would interact to a greater degree with the π-electron system, of the heterocyclic ring than would a nitro group substituted in the 5-position. On examination of a range of 2-nitroimidazoles originally synthesised by Roche Products, one such compound Ro-07-0582, or misonidazole, was found to be a very efficient sensitizer both <u>in vitro</u> and <u>in vivo</u>[8,9].

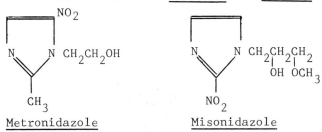

Metronidazole   Misonidazole

Figure 2 illustrates the sensitizing ability of misonidazole in X-irradiated hypoxic Chinese Hamster cells[11]. Clearly, in hypoxia, appreciable sensitization at 1 mM is observed and at 10 mM the sensitization is comparable to that shown by oxygen itself.

Figure 3 shows data[12] on the sensitizing efficiency of miso-nidazole <u>in vitro</u> collected from several published studies. Both for metronidazole and misonidazole the data points do not

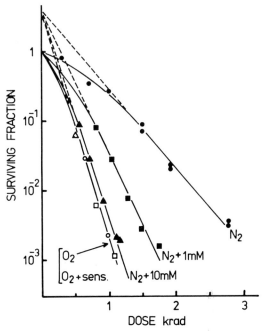

Fig. 2. Sensitization of hypoxic Chinese Hamster cells by misonidazole (ref. 11).

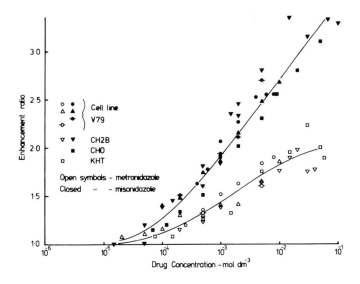

Fig. 3. Sensitization of a variety of cell lines by misonidazole and metronidazole (ref. 12).

show much scatter indicating that, at least for these cell lines, the sensitizing efficiencies of both drugs are fairly constant.

There are now many _in vivo_ studies of the sensitizing ability of metronidazole and particularly misonidazole in experimental tumour systems. Almost all these show pronounced sensitization when the drug is given before irradiation. Figure 4 shows the effect of misonidazole on the tumour control probabilities for the anaplastic MT tumour implanted in an inbred strain of WHT/Ht mice[13].

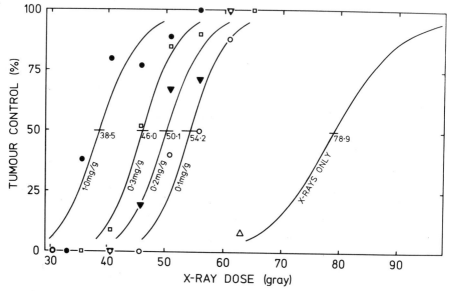

Fig. 4. Radiation sensitization of MT tumours by misonidazole at 1 mg/g (●), 0.3mg/g (□), 0.2mg/g (▼) and 0.1mg/g (o). X-rays alone (x) (ref.13).

The mice were given various concentrations of misonidazole 30 minutes before X-irradiation. The displacement of the 80 day TCD_{50} control value from 78.9 gray to 38.5 gray with increasing drug concentration indicates considerable sensitization. The calculated enhancement ratios or dose reduction factors are 1.46 (0.1 mg/g), 1.57 (0.2 mg/g), 1.17 (0.3 mg/g) and 2.05 (1.0 mg/g).

The large enhancement ratios found for single dose treatments with X-rays and misonidazole would be expected to be smaller when the drug is given with multiple fractions of radiation spaced over a period, due to re-oxygenation processes reducing the hypoxic cell fraction.   Numerous fractionation studies of this type have been carried out with misonidazole (collected papers in ref.14).   An interesting result[15] showing that sensitization can occur in the MT tumour even with 20 fraction treatments is shown in Figure 5.

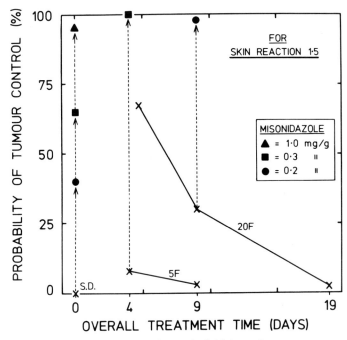

Fig. 5. Dependence of control probability for MT tumours X-irradiated after administration of misonidazole (see text) (ref. 15).

The Figure shows the tumour control probability of MT tumours treated with either single doses of radiation, 5 fractions in 4 or 9 days and 20 fractions in 4, 9 and 19 days.   The mice were given 0.2, 0.3 of 1.0 mg/g with single radiation doses, 0.3 mg/g with each fraction of the 5 fraction treatments and 0.2 mg/g with each fraction of the 20 fraction treatments.   Control probabilities for each schedule were measured for the X-ray dose that would produce a constant level of skin damage (for details see reference). For X-rays alone, 20 fractions are better than 5 fractions for this tumour provided overall treatment time did not exceed 19 days. However, misonidazole improved both schedules to a uniform high level. This result suggests that by taking the criticality out of the choice of fractionation schedule, optimum therapy might be achievable clinically even though the fractionation schedule alone would not be optimum. With some other experimental tumour systems, however, the advantage afforded by misonidazole can become smaller with some fractionation schedules (see papers in ref.14).

HYPOXIC CYTOTOXICITY OF MISONIDAZOLE

There is now much evidence[14] that in the absence of radiation, misonidazole and similar nitro-containing compounds are much more toxic to hypoxic compared with oxic mammalian cells. Figure 6 shows some _in vitro_ data demonstrating the effect in hypoxic cultures of Chinese Hamster cells. Oxic cells survive 5 mM misonidazole for almost 3 days before they begin to lose viability. However, in anoxia, misonidazole is highly toxic. The drug dose-time responses generally show an initial shoulder region followed by an exponential region (not clearly evident for the time scale in Fig. 6). Increase of drug dose causes both a reduction in the shoulder and an increase in the slope. The mechanism of this toxicity is believed to be associated with the production of a toxic substance following anaerobic metabolism of the drug[14]. There is now good evidence that this hypoxic cytotoxicity is due to processes other than those involved in hypoxic cell radiosensitization. For example, efficiency of sensitization _in vitro_ shows little dependence on temperature yet the hypoxic toxicity in cells treated with misonidazole in the absence of radiation is very temperature-

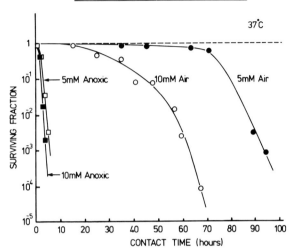

Fig. 6. The cytotoxic effect of misonidazole towards hypoxic and aerobic mammalian cells (ref. 12).

dependent. The question whether this cytotoxic effect can occur in human tumours has an important bearing on the possible future role of these drugs in combination with other cytotoxic drugs for the treatment of metastatic disease, in addition to their use in radiotherapy.

Pre-incubation effects of misonidazole

A phenomenon possibly related to the hypoxic cytotoxic properties of misonidazole is the potentiation of cellular damage by pre-incubation of hypoxic cells with the drug prior to exposure to radiation, heat or cytotoxic drugs.

Whitmore and colleagues[16] reported that if hypoxic cells are exposed to misonidazole for three hours and the cells are then irradiated after the drug has been removed by successive washing, the hypoxic survival curve shows a complete loss of the shoulder. In our laboratory[17] we have found that overnight incubation of hypoxic V79 cells with only 60µg/ml (0.3 mM) misonidazole followed by drug removal and irradiation in hypoxia, also shows a complete suppression of the shoulder of the survival curve. This drug concentration is in the range of clinical tolerance and the shoulder suppression effect, if applicable to hypoxic cells in human tumours, could have a profound influence on radiation response to multifraction radiotherapy irrespective of any <u>direct</u> sensitization of hypoxic cells by misonidazole.

Recently, we have found that pre-incubation of hypoxic V79 cells to misonidazole followed by drug removal, also makes the cells much more sensitive to heat and the effects of some cytotoxic drugs, e.g. melphalan[17]. Any possible relevance of these findings to future treatment remains to be seen.

CLINICAL INVESTIGATIONS WITH MISONIDAZOLE
Early studies

The evidence from mouse tumours led to pilot studies of misonidazole as a radiation sensitizer in man, particularly since evidence of radiation-sensitization of human gliomas by metronidazole had previously been observed by Urtasun and colleagues[10]. Some of the criteria necessary for consideration of sensitizers for clinical use would appear to be met by misonidazole. The fact that this class of sensitizer acts only against hypoxic cells indicates that radiation damage to normal tissue which is usually well-oxygenated, should not be enhanced. In this respect, therefore, misonidazole is tumour specific. Early studies showed that both metronidazole and misonidazole are fairly well tolerated in single doses[18] and there is also much evidence of tumour penetration by misonidazole.

Evidence of sensitization was obtained from preliminary single radiation dose studies in man. Potentiation of radiation effect was noted in normal skin made artifically hypoxic[19] and studies of the radiation response of tumour nodules, some treated with,

some without, misonidazole, showed evidence of increased effect[20].
Phase 1 studies are now complete and randomised controlled trials
designed to show conclusive evidence of clinical benefit, are in
progress for various tumour sites.

Neurotoxicity

Although the radiobiological data and the preliminary clinical
data from single dose studies are promising, it is now clear that
misonidazole is neurotoxic.   Some patients receiving multiple
doses of misonidazole develop a sensory peripheral neuropathy
towards the end of, or shortly after, treatment.   The incidence
is sharply dose-dependent and Dische[21] has recommended that the
total dose should not excees $12g/m^2$.   Since the drug dose given
with each individual radiation fraction will clearly depend on
the total number of fractions given, choice of fractionation
regimes will be important in clinical trials with misonidazole.

Clinical trials

Several options are available in the design of clinical
trials with misonidazole.   For example, the drug could be used
with: a) every fraction of a conventional small-fraction regime
such as 20-30 fractions in 4-6 weeks, b) with every fraction of
a regime employing a small number of fractions, or c) with some
but not all fractions of a given regime (such as one investigated
by Bleehen[22], 12F/4 weeks with the drug given once weekly with
a larger radiation fraction).   The human dosage of misonidazole
is limited ultimately by its neurotoxicity and it is clear that
this will prevent the drug from being used at a level necessary
for the maximum degree of sensitization theoretically possible,
i.e. the full value of the oxygen enhancement ratio whatever
fractionation is used.   Figure 7 shows the enhancement ratio
for sensitization of hypoxic Chinese Hamster cells as a function
of the concentration in the medium.   The proposition that such

a curve might apply to sensitization of human tumours rests on two main assumptions: a) the sensitization efficiency of misonidazole is not reduced for hypoxic cells _in vivo_ compared to those _in vitro_, and b) the concentration of the drug in hypoxic tumour cells is similar to that measured in the serum at the same time. Both these assumptions appear to be justifiable. It has been shown in mouse tumours that the sensitizing efficiency of misonidazole is at least as high as that measured _in vitro_. Further, there is much evidence on the satisfactory penetration of misonidazole into human tumours.

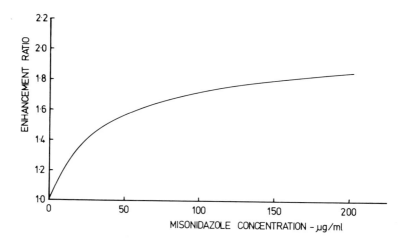

Fig. 7. Radiation sensitization of Chinese Hamster cells by misonidazole. Dependence of enhancement ratio on misonidazole concentration (from ref. 11).

Since the recommended maximum total dose should not exceed $12g/m^2$, the drug dose per fraction will obviously depend on the total number of fractions. This suggests that more benefit might be obtainable with unconventional fractionation regimes using a relatively small number of large fraction sizes. This is one direction to pursue, certainly. However, the implications of hypoxic cytotoxicity and related phenomena must be taken into account. For this reason alone, it is correct that some misonidazole trials are being carried out with fairly conventional regimens.

Various prospective randomised trials of misonidazole with radiotherapy are in progress. Sealy[23] is using six equal fractions over three weeks to treat advanced head and neck cancer. Misonidazole ($12g/m^2$) is given with each radiation fraction of 600 rads. Dische and Saunders (private communication) are also investigating this treatment regime for treatment of Ca bronchus. Urtasun in a development from his metronidazole trial is using misonidazole with 9 equal fractions of radiation in three weeks for treating glioblasoma. In this trial, the control arm is conventional 6 weeks treatment. Other investigations are in progress.[15] In particular, phase 1 studies are complete in the United States and phase 11 studies are in progress for a variety of tumour sites and protocols. In the United Kingdom, the Medical Research Council, in collaboration with Roche Products Ltd., have set up three co-operative studies of misonidazole:

a) Glioblastoma treated with 20F/4W to a total dose of 4500 rads with 20 equal doses of misonidazole (total $12g/m^2$);

b) Ca cervix III treated over four weeks with 20 equal fractions to 4250 rads followed by 3500 rads to Pt A. Misonidazole is given in 24 equal fractions (total $12g/m^2$).

c) Cancer of the head and neck region treated with 10 fractions over 3 weeks to 4500 rads with 10 equal fractions of $1.2g/m^2$ misonidazole.

A recent finding that may have considerable implications in reducing neurotoxicity concerns the effect of phenytoin on the pharmacokinetics of misonidazole. Independently, Bleehen and Workman in the U.K., and Phillips, Wasserman and co-workers in the U.S. (private communications) have found that patients receiving phenytoin show a marked reduction in the half-life of misonidazole although the peak levels are unchanged. A similar effect is observed in laboratory mice. Since the neurotoxicity of misonidazole in man is likely to be a function of total tissue exposure to the drug, reduction in half-life without reduction in peak levels could increase the therapeutic ratio considerably.

DEVELOPMENT OF NEW DRUGS

The toxicity of misonidazole will prevent its use clinically at doses necessary for maximum sensitization. New drugs with better therapeutic ratios are required therefore. Many compounds are known which show appreciable sensitizing properties in vitro and there is no reason to suppose that the limit of efficiency in vivo has been attained with the only two drugs that have reached the clinical stage, i.e. metronidazole and misonidazole. It is true that the requirements for sensitization of solid tumours in vivo disqualify many compounds that are otherwise very active as sensitizers in vitro. Nevertheless, structure activity studies using cellular systems in vitro have been most useful in establishing some of the guidelines for the development of new drugs. Indeed, several new compounds have been identified with sensitizing efficiencies in vitro considerably greater than that of misonidazole.

The most important factor affecting sensitization efficiency is the electron affinity of the compound. This property is associated with the ability of a molecule to act as an oxidizing agent or electron sink at the radiation chemical level and is possessed by oxygen and many other chemical compounds. The higher the electron affinity of the compound, the greater is the sensitizing efficiency expressed in terms of the concentration required for a given amount of sensitization. Electron affinity correlations have been most useful in developing new sensitizers[24]. However, data on the relative efficacies of different compounds are of limited value unless the appropriate information relevant to their toxic properties is also available. At the present time, one of the highest priorities is to obtain knowledge of the various structural, chemical, physical and biological characteristics of the sensitizers which might confer undesirable neurotoxic properties on these compounds. Drug-induced damage to the peripheral nervous system in laboratory animals is susceptible to laboratory investigation and has been studied extensively for other types of drugs. Several test systems employing behavioural, morphological and biochemical endpoints are currently in use to investigate the neurotoxicity of misonidazole and related compounds. Of possible significance is the observation of demyelination in peripheral nerve fibres of patients treated with misonidazole during radiotherapy[25]. Similarly, demyelination and axonal degeneration has been observed in peripheral nerves of mice treated with misonidazole[26] Experimental studies of this and other types may prove useful as a prescreen in the study of sensitizers with the aim of establish-ing the physical and chemical properties of sensitizers associated with neurotoxicity. For example, if it transpired that demyelination is linked to the lipophilic properties of the sensi-tizers, this information would be most useful in the design of new drugs since lipophilicity does not appear greatly to affect sensitizing efficiency, at least _in vitro._

REFERENCES

1. Thomlinson, R.H. and Gray, L.H. (1955) Brit. J. Cancer, 9, 539-549.

2. Adams, G.E. and Dewey, D.L. (1963) Biochem. Biophys. Res. Commun., 12, 473-477.

3. Adams, G.E. and Cooke, M.S. (1969) Int. J. Radiat. Biol., 15, 457-471.

4. Chapman, J.D., Webb, R.G. and Borsa, J. (1971) Int. J. Radiat. Biol., 19, 561-574.

5. Adams, G.E., Asquith, J.C., Dewey, D.L., Foster, J.L., Michael, B.D. and Willson, R.L. (1971) Int. J. Radiat. Biol., 575-585.

6. Chapman, J.D., Reuvers, A.P., Borsa, J., Petkau, A. and McCalla, D.R. (1972) Cancer Res., 32, 2616-2624.

7. Foster, J.L. and Willson, R.L. (1973) Brit. J. Radiol., 6, 234-235.

8. Adams, G.E. (1977) Hypoxic cell sensitizers for radiotherapy in "Cancer: A Comprehensive Treatise" Vol.6 ed. R.F.Becker, Plenum Press, New York, pp.181-223.

9. Fowler, J.F. and Denekamp, J. (1979).A Review of Hypoxic Cell Radiosensitization in Experimental Tumours in Pharmacology and Therapeutics, Pergamon Press (in press).

10. Urtasun, R.C., Band, P., Chapman, J.D., Feldstein, M.C., Mielke, B. and Fryer, C. (1976) N. Engl. J. Med., 294, 1364-1367.

11. Asquith, J.C., Watts, M.E., Patel, K.B., Smithen, C.E. and Adams, G.E. (1974) Radiation Research, 60, 108-118.

12. Stratford, I.J. (1979) in "Radiosensitizers of Hypoxic Cells", Elsevier-North Holland, pp.109-128.

13. Sheldon, P.W. and Hill, S.A. (1977) Brit. J. Cancer 35, 795-808 (and private communication).

14. Collected papers in "Hypoxic Cell Sensitizers in Radiobiology and Radiotherapy", Brit. J. Cancer (1978) 37, Suppl. III, pp.1-321.

15. Sheldon, P.W. and Fowler, J.F. (1978) Brit. J. Cancer, 37, Supple.III, 242-245.

16. Whitmore, G.F., Gulyas, S. and Varghese, A.J. (1978) Brit. J. Cancer 37, Suppl.III, 115-119.

17. Rajaratnam, S., Kandaiya, S., Stratford, I.J. and Adams, G.E. (unpublished).

18. Gray, A.J., Dische, S., Adams, G.E., Flockhart, I.R. and Foster, J.L. (1976) Clin. Radiol., 27, 151-157.

19. Dische, S., Gray, A.J. and Zanelli, G.D. (1976) Clin. Radiol., 27, 159-166.

20. Thomlinson, R.H., Dische, S., Gray, A.J. and Errington, L.M. (1976) Clin. Radiol. 27, 167-174.

21. Saunders, M.I., Dische, S., Anderson, P. and Flockhart, I.R. (1978) Brit. J. Cancer, 37, Suppl.III, 268-270.

22. Wiltshire, C.R., Workman, P., Watson, J.V. and Bleehen, N.M. (1978) Brit. J. Cancer, 37, Suppl.III, 286-289.

23. Sealy, R. (1978) Brit. J. Cancer, 37, Suppl.III, 314-317.

24. Adams, G.E., Clarke, E.D., Flockhart, I.R., Jacobs, R.S., Sehmi, D.S., Stratford, I.J., Wardman, P. and Watts, M.E. (1979) Int. J. Rad. Biol., 35, 133-150, and references therein.

25. Urtasun, R.C., Chapman, J.D., Feldstein, M.C., Band, R.P., Rabin, H.R., Wilson, A.F., Marynowski, B., Starreveld, E. and Shnitka, T. (1978) Brit. J. Cancer, 37, Suppl.III, 271-275.

26. Adams, G.E., Dawson, K.B. and Stratford, I.J. In Proc. Int. Meeting for Radio-Oncology, May 1978, Vienna, Georg Thieme, Stuttgart (in press).

© 1979, Elsevier/North-Holland Biomedical Press
Treatment of Radioresistant Cancers
M. Abe, K. Sakamoto and T.L. Phillips eds.

TREATMENT OF RADIORESISTANT TUMORS: A CRITERION OF CHOICE BETWEEN
CONVENTIONAL AND NON-CONVENTIONAL RADIOTHERAPY IN COMBINATION
WITH HYPERTHERMIA AND/OR MISONIDAZOLE.

GIORGIO ARCANGELI[1], FRANCESCO MAURO[2], CARLO NERVI[1] and MARIA CHIA-
RA PARDINI[1-2]
[1]Istituto Medico Scientifico, Clinica Villa Flaminia, 00191 Rome,
and [2]Laboratorio di Dosimetria e Biofisica, Comitato Nazionale
Energia Nucleare, 00100 Rome, (Italy)

INTRODUCTION

The radioresistance of a tumor is the clinical outcome resulting
from a variety of phenomena overlapping at the cellular and tissu-
lar level. In the past, several approaches have been suggested in
the attempt to cope with such a problem. These approaches have be-
en demonstrated to be either unsatisfactory (e.g., hyperboric oxygen, halogenated pyrimidines) or anyhow involving a high level of
technological complexity (e.g., particle beam therapy).

More recently, several multimodality treatments became available
in clinical practice after the introduction of chemical radiosensitizers[1], supposedly specific for hypoxic cells, and local hyperthermia[2], particularly effective on S-phase and/or hypoxic cells.
In several cases, in fact, the fraction of hypoxic cells has been
often indicated as the main responsible of tumor radioresistance.
The degree of involvement of clonogenic non-proliferating cells
and of "intrinsically" radioresistant cells in determining a poor
radiation response is still largely unknown.

PROPAEDEUTIC CLINICAL OBSERVATIONS

Our previous experience[3] on treating with different modalities
patients with multiple (N_2-N_3) neck node metastases from head and
neck (H&N) cancer has been definitively positive. The results are
encouraging in spite of the fact that the data concern the immedia
te local response with a follow-up of 4-6 months only and have be-
en collected and compared by treating with different modalities
different lesions of the same patients. These clinical results indicate the effectiveness, in respect to a hystorical series of pa-

tients treated with conventional fractionation (2 Gy/day, 5 days/
week), of either multiple daily fractionation (MDF) alone (2+1.5+
1.5 Gy/day, 5 days/week) or MDF + Hyperthermia (500 MHz, 42°- 43°
C,45 min.,after the 2nd daily fraction, on day 1, 3 and 5 of each
week) or MDF + Misonidazole (1.2 g/m^2 daily, 2 h before the first
fraction, up to a maximum dose of 12 g/m^2) or MDF + Hyperthermia
+ Misonidazole. The latter modality appears to be possibly the
most effective and inducing in 80% of lesions a complete local tumor response lasting longer in time, at least within the limits of
the follow-up.

This approach can be considered preliminarly satisfactory when
carried out on cases in advanced stages of disease and with multiple lesions. However, considering that all these combinations of
modalities are time-consuming and difficult to be carried out on a
large number of randomized cases, the problem arises on how to se-
lect the best treatment modality according to the individual tumor
characteristics. At the present stage, preceding that of a full
randomized trial, this means the identification of the radioresistant tumors prior to the treatment

Unfortunately, at present, no biological property or pathological feature is known to be a clear-cut predictor of radiation response. In recent years, our clinical research group has carried
out a particular effort in looking out for a meaningful predictor
or at least such that a "biological stratification" could be attempted. Until now this research has not been fruitful from a
practical point of view, as summarized in Table 1.

Recently, Holsti, Salmo and Elkind[6] proposed, although in a different context pursuing the exploitation of a possible increase in
reoxygenation, the use of (an) initial large fractional dose(s) of
radiation. In particular, in patients with lung metastases or non-
oat cell lung carcinoma, they observed that the tumor shrinkage
could be used to distinguish a well reacting from a poorly reacting group. The presence of two types of radiation response could
be often recognized one week after a single 10 Gy dose and could
not be explained in terms of histology or size.

TABLE 1

POSSIBLE PREDICTOR	RELATION TO RESPONSE
Tumor stage (or size)	Recognizable but difficult to quantify or in some cases (e.g., H&N), absent[4]
Growth rate Generation time Growth fraction	Scarce but often unreliable[4]
Presence of single vs. multiple cell populations	None[5]
Fraction of hypoxic cells	? (At present not detectable before treatment)
Fraction of non-proliferating cells	? (Detectable, but their radiation response characteristics are still under discussion)

On these bases, we decided to test the possibility of employing a large initial fractional dose as a rough predictor of radiation response. This approach implies the assumption that the response to such dose reflects the actual cell killing resulting from the presence of several subpopulations of different radiosensitivity.

MATERIALS AND METHODS

Patients

34 patients with advanced or large recurrent tumors were selected for this study: 10 patients with postoperative pelvic recurrences from rectal cancer (adenocarcinomata), 15 with head and neck primaries (squamous cell, 10 grade III and 5 grade IV) and 9 with bladder tumors (transitional cell, 6 grade III and 3 grade IV). Before undergoing therapy patients were accurately studied with C.A.T., barium enema, cystoscopy or retrograde cystography, and/or physical examination in order to assess the volume of the lesions. The same examinations were repeated 10 days after the initial radiation fraction in order to estimate the percent tumor shrinkage as accurately as possible. Patients previously treated with radiotherapy or chemotherapy did not enter the study.

Irradiation

All patients treated with 5.7 MeV photons from a Neptune Linear Accelerator by means of two parallel opposing fields or arc therapy, received a first radiation fraction of 8-10 Gy depending on the volume and the particular region treated. After 10 days, patients were accurately revaluated to assess the initial tumor shrinkage and then on day 11 they began the conventional fractionation course of radiotherapy of 2 Gy/day, 5 days/week, up to a total of 60-75 Gy. Patients not showing a marked shrinkage at the end of treatment underwent chemotherapy or when possible radical surgery.

RESULTS

10 days after receiving an initial fractional dose of 8-10 Gy, patients were classified as responders or non-responders according to the degree of tumor shrinkage. The tumors considered as not responding were those exhibiting increase of growth, no shrinking, or shrinking within 10% only.

The results after the initial dose are summarized in Table 2. They show that in all sites with no striking differences among sites, 44-60% of tumors could be classified as responding, the rate of shrinkage being 10 to 50%.

TABLE 2
PATIENTS RESPONDING TO THE INITIAL FRACTIONAL
RADIATION DOSE (8-10 Gy) (sites)

H&N	8/15	53%
BLADDER	4/9	44%
RECTAL RECURR.	6/10	60%
total	18/34	53%

The same data were analyzed according to tumor hystology, as reported in Table 3. Once again, at the present level of statistical significance, no difference could be detected between tumors of different histology, the range of responders being 33 to 60%.

TABLE 3

PATIENTS RESPONDING TO THE INITIAL FRACTIONAL
RADIATION DOSE 48-10 Gy) (Hystology & grading)

SQUAMOUS	grade III	5/10	50%
	grade IV	3/5	60%
TRANSITIONAL	grade III	3/6	50%
	grade IV	1/3	33%
ADENOCARC.		6/10	53%
		18/34	53%

The results of the remaining part of radiotherapy are shown in
Table 4 only for the patients classified as responders. This is be
cuase none of the non responding patients exhibited a complete response (that is 100% shrinkage) at the end of treatment or by 10
days thereafter. On the contrary, as evidenced by table 4, the majority of responding patients exhibited a complete response. In
fact only 25% to 33% of the responding tumors did not exhibit a
complete response by the end of treatment.

TABLE 4

RESULTS (COMPLETE RESPONSE) OF CONVENTIONAL
RADIOTHERAPY IN PATIENTS RESPONDING TO THE
INITIAL FRACTIONAL RADIATION DOSE (8-10 Gy)
(Sites)

H&N	6/8	75%
BLADDER	3/4	75%
RECTAL RECURR.	4/6	67%

The same data are analyzed according to tumor histology in Table
5, suggesting that there are no grading differences such that the
failures of prediction could be explained.

TABLE 5

RESULTS (COMPLETE RESPONSE) OF CONVENTIONAL RADIOTHERAPY IN
PATIENTS RESPONDING TO THE INITIAL FRACTIONAL RADIATION DOSE
(8-10 Gy) (Hystology & grading)

SQUAMOUS	grade III	4/5	80%
	grade IV	2/3	67%
TRANSITIONAL	grade III	2/3	67%
	grade IV	1/1	100%
ADENOCARC.		4/6	67%

DISCUSSION

The present results show that after an initial large fractional radiation dose some tumors exhibited a shrinkage greater than 10%. The majority of these tumors underwent complete local response fol lowing conventional fractionation radiotherapy, indicating that, although some "false positive" could be observed, the probability of predicting a complete response is fairly high at least in tumors under study. However, none of the tumors not responding to the initial fractional radiation dose exhibited a complete local response following conventional fractionation. In other words no "false negative" could be observed and the prediction of incomplete responses could be considered very reliable. Such a strategy allows the selection of a well defined patient population, with tumors characterized by resistant cellular components, to be directly and satisfactory destined to particular treatment modalities. This kind of "biological stratification" for individualized treatment selection is at present under study. Our strategy is complete ly described in Table 6.

TABLE 6

I.M.S. PROTOCOL

day 1   8-10 Gy initial fraction

day 2 to 9   rest

day 10   observation

GOOD RESPONSE   POOR RESPONSE

"radiosensitive"   "radioresistant"

(hypoxic cell fraction)

(oxygenation?)   (no reoxygenation?)

CONVENTIONAL   MDF
FRACTIONATION   1.8+1.8+1.8 Gy/day,

(or MDF?)   4 h interval

+

HYPERTHERMIA (~ 43°C)
30-40 min exposure, immediately after 2nd daily fraction, each other day

and/or

MISONIDAZOLE
1.2 g/m^2, 2 h before 1st dai
ly fraction, up to a total
dose of 12 g/m^2

Our data also show that hystology grading does not affect the response to the initial large fractional dose, being therefore of no value in predicting local tumor response. The size of the initial dose fraction has been decided on a purely empiric ground considering that, by giving about one sixth to one eighth of the whole dose in a single fraction, the chances of late radiation effects would be not relevantly increased, while the initial cell killing could be quite relevant to indicate the presence of "radioresistant" cell compartments.

REFERENCES

1. Adams, G.E., Fowler, J.F. and Wardmann,P., eds.(1978) Hypoxic Cell Sensitizers in Radiobiology and Radiotherapy, The British Journal of Cancer, Supplement No.III, pp. 1-321.

2. Streffer,C. et al., eds. (1978) Cancer Therapy by Hyperthermia and Radiation, Urban & Schwarzenberg, Baltimore-Münich, pp. 1-344.

3. Arcangeli, G., Barocas, A., Mauro, F., Nervi, C., Spanò, M., Tabocchini, A. (1979) Cancer, in press.

4. Nervi, C., Arcangeli, G., Badaracco, G., Cortese, M., Morelli, M., and Starace, G. (1978) Cancer, 41, 900-906.

5. Nervi, C., Badaracco, G., Morelli, M., and Starace, G. (1979) Cancer (in press).

6. Holsti, L.R., Salmo, M., and Elkind,M.M. (1978) Brit. J. Cancer, 37, Suppl. III, 307-310.

HYPOXIC CELL SENSITIZER STUDIES IN THE UNITED STATES

THEODORE L. PHILLIPS, M.D.

Department of Radiation Oncology, University of California, M-330, San Francisco,
California, 94143 (USA)

TODD H. WASSERMAN, M.D.

Division of Radiation Oncology, Mallinckrodt Institute of Radiology, Washington
University School of Medicine, 4511 Forest Park Boulevard, St. Louis, Missouri,
63108 (USA)

ABSTRACT

The study of the hypoxic cell sensitizer misonidazole began in the United
States through the Radiation Therapy Oncology Group in June 1977. A total of
104 patients was accessioned into a Phase I study which evaluated the pharmacology and toxicity of the drug and established maximum tolerated doses. This
study revealed that toxicity included not only peripheral neuropathy, nausea and
vomiting, but also central nervous system effects including ototoxicity and encephalopathy. The maximum tolerated dose appeared to be 12 gm/m^2 in 3 weeks and
15 gm/m^2 in 6 weeks. Subsequent Phase II studies have revealed that these doses
must be reduced to 10 and 12 gm/m^2, respectively, in patients with head and neck
cancer, lung cancer, and other sites because of increased sensitivity to the
drug. Although none of the studies were designed to specifically measure efficacy, observations of patients with multiple lesions treated with and without
misonidazole suggest effective sensitization in patients with squamous cell carcinomas.

INTRODUCTION

Following the introduction of misonidazole experimentally, it was entered into Phase I clinical trials first in the United Kingdom and then in Canada.[1,2]
Based on the data available from these studies, it was clear that the drug had
significant hypoxic cell sensitizing capabilities and was reasonably well tolerated clinically, with the major side effect considered to be peripheral sensory
neuropathy. Based on this information a Phase I clinical study was started in
June 1977 by the Radiation Therapy Oncology Group (RTOG) under the auspices of
the National Cancer Institute.[3] This Phase I study was conducted at the University of California, San Francisco, and Roswell Park Memorial Institute, Buffalo,
New York. It was designed to study in depth the toxicity to be expected from
misonidazole and to establish maximum tolerated doses for various drug administration schemes, including once, twice, and three times weekly administration
and, in certain cases, daily administration. It was also designed to measure

the pharmacologic distribution of the drug, its excretion, and the nature of the neuropathies to be observed.

In July 1978 the first of a series of Phase II studies was opened by the RTOG. These studies are designed to evaluate misonidazole in a specific disease site using a specific drug dose schedule and a specific radiation schedule. They are designed to determine the tolerance of the patients in this particular disease group to the drug dosage prescribed and to establish the nature of the radiation effects on the tumor and normal tissues prior to designing randomized Phase III studies. This paper will review the results of these studies as of April 1979.

Phase I Study

All patients entered in the Phase I study had advanced solid tumors not amenable to conventional therapy and were candidates for palliative local radiotherapy. All patients had recovered from any effects of prior chemotherapy and had normal renal, bone marrow and liver function. A few patients had minor liver enzyme elevations. All patients had signed approved informed consent forms. All patients were treated at only one drug dose level with no dose escalation in a given patient. Two patients had a repeated course; this will be detailed later. The drug was given as an enteric, coated 0.5 gm tablet after a light breakfast, or recently as 0.5 gm and 0.1 gm capsules. Radiation therapy was given 4-6 hrs after drug administration to allow for maximum serum and tumor tissue levels. All patients had pharmacological evaluation with blood levels drawn at the time of radiation, and most patients in the earlier phase of the study had serial blood and urine determinations with pharmacology curves. Pharmacology was done via UV spectrophotometry or high pressure liquid chromatography.

TABLE 1

MISONIDAZOLE PHASE I STUDY

Schema of Patient Entry by Dose Level and Number of Doses

Gm/m^2	Weekly doses	Total dose gm/m^2	No. patients	Incomplete Patients*		
				D	W	ND
1.0	3	3	3	–	–	––
2.0	3	6	4	–	–	––
3.0	3	9	4	1	–	1
4.0	3	12	3	1	–	––
5.0	3	15	4	–	2	––
1.0	6	6	3	1	1	––
2.0	6	12	9	1	1	2
2.5	6	15	5	–	2	––
3.0	6	18	5	–	5	––
	149 Drug Doses		40 pts.	4	11	3

*D=premature death; W=patient withdrawal; ND=lack of drug.

A weekly dose schedule was used in the first phase of the study. The schema is presented in Table 1. All patients received weekly doses for 3 or 6 weeks. Patients are listed as incomplete if they received one or more doses but did not complete the planned dose schedule; the reasons for this are indicated in the Table. The initial dose was escalated to 5 gm/m^2 for 3 weeks and 3 gm/m^2 for 6 weeks. Because frequency of administration is important in scheduling with radiation, further exploration of higher dose levels was deemed not as important as investigation of more frequent dose schedules, and thus further dose escalation was not done on the weekly schedule. The additional Phase I schema listed in Table 2 was used in the second part of the study. This investigated 2 and 3 times per week schedules and some daily schedules. Forty patients were entered into the initial part of the study on the weekly dose schedule and 64 in the additional Phase I schema, for a total of 104 patients.

TABLE 2

ADDITIONAL PHASE I SCHEMA

Dose schedule	Dose gm/m^2	Total dose gm/m^2	No. pts. entered	No. completed
3X/wk X 3 wks	2.0	12	12	10
(6 doses)	2.5	15	6	4
3X/wk X 6 wks	1.25	15	14	10
(12 doses)	1.5	18	6	2
	1.75	21	1	1
3X/wk X 2 wks	1.5	9	2	2
(6 doses)				
3X/wk X $2^1/_3$ wks	1.5	10.5	3	3
(7 doses)	1.75	12.25	4	2
Once/day X 5 days	1.5	7.5	6	6
(5 doses)				
Once/day X 7 days	1.5	10.5	6	3
(7 doses)	1.75	12.25	4	2
			64	45

The individual doses ranged from 1 - 5 gm/m^2 and sera levels were proportional to the dose given (shown in Table 3). The dose, number of determinations, and the mean 4 - 6 hour serum level in µg/ml of both misonidazole (Ro-07-0582) and desmethylmisonidazole (Ro-05-9963), the principle metabolite, are shown with the standard deviations. Emphasis was placed on the 4-6 hour serum level, as this reflected the level at the time of radiation. The range of time reflects the inability to precisely schedule the radiation at a certain time point. The mean level reflects the average of all the 4-6 hour levels for all doses given for a given patient. The values obtained for 0582 and 9963 were added together, as only the HPLC method separates the 2 species--the UV method does not. The mean 4-6 hour level of both species was felt to be the best value to be considered for further evaluation in Phase II studies. Peak sera levels tend to be higher, but were not chosen because without doing complete pharmacologic serum half-life curves the peak levels would not be known. Peak sera levels tend to occur at 2-3 hours, with some plateau up to the 4-6 hour period. Half-life determinations in the initial 33 patients ranged from 3-25 hours, with a mean of 15 hours and a median of 14 hours.

TABLE 3

MISONIDAZOLE PHASE I STUDY

Relationship of Dose to Mean 4-6 Hour Serum Level

Dose gm/m^2	No. of doses (determinations)	Mean 4-6 hr serum level (µg/ml) (0582 + 9963)	± Standard deviation of:
1.0	17	30	± 9
1.25	116	46	± 6
1.5	46	54	±17
1.75	12	61	±10
2.0	86	76	±14
2.5	43	98	±23
3.0	25	116	±26
4.0	8	175	±56
5.0	7	183	±60

The urine excretion is principally of the active metabolite desmethylmisonidazole. Of 16 patients who had urinary measurements, the total percent excretion of both species in 24 hours ranged from 12 - 65%, with a mean of 28% and a median of 23%. Twenty-four hour stool levels were essentially nil, including 1 patient with liver dysfunction. We feel that the unaccounted for percentage is probably present in the urine or stool as smaller species, not detected by the assay used. Tumor biopsies were done in 2 patients and were 80% and 90% of the peak sera levels. A pleural fluid sample taken at 6 hours from one patient was 100% of the simultaneous blood level. The pharmacologic study has established the good absorption, bio-availability, general body distribution, and pharmacological stability characteristics of the drug.

When the patient doses (expressed in gm/m^2) and the patient blood levels (expressed in µg/ml) are compared to enhancement ratios seen in experimental studies in vitro and in vivo, as summarized by McNally et al.[4], good evidence of enhancement is seen. Studies of experimental tumors by McNally[4] and human skin experiments by Dische et al.[5] support enhancement ratios which range from 1.25

at approximately 20 µg/ml to approximately 1.75 at 100 µg/ml. One exception is the result reported by Johnson et al.[6] in which enhancement of the sensitivity of hypoxic skin in primates was only 1.3 at 100 µg/ml.

In the Phase I RTOG study, a dose of 1 gm/m^2 resulted in a blood level of 30 µg/ml which would produce an enhancement ratio of approximately 1.35. Likewise, a drug dose of 1.25 gm/m^2 resulted in a blood level of 46 µg/ml with an expected enhancement ratio of approximately 1.45; 1.5 gm/m^2 of drug resulted in a blood level of 54 µg/ml with an expected enhancement ratio of approximately 1.5; and a drug dose of 2 gm/m^2 resulted in a blood level of 76 µg/ml with an expected enhancement ratio of about 1.65. Thus it would appear that the doses achievable clinically will produce enhancement ratios between 1.3 and 1.7. This degree of enhancement should be detectable in randomized clinical trials.

Patients were carefully monitored with repeated histories, physicals, and blood tests for bone marrow, renal, liver and other toxicities. It is important to note that no renal, liver, or bone marrow toxicity was observed. The principle toxicities consisted of acute nausea and vomiting and delayed cumulative neurotoxicity.

Acute nausea and vomiting occurred in about one-fourth of the patients, usually within 1-12 hours after the drug dose and often at the time of or soon after the radiation. It may be related both to the gastrointestinal effects of the drug and often to additive radiation induced nausea. It was somewhat dose related in that patients at higher drug dose levels had a higher tendency toward toxicity. This may be related to the number of tablets that the patient is required to swallow, and another dose formulation might decrease this toxicity. The nausea and vomiting was somewhat ameliorated by pre-treatment administration of anti-emetics, compazine suppository 25 mg 1 hr before drug dose, and this has become a standard drug administration procedure.

The dose limiting toxicity for repeated doses was neurotoxicity, primarily a peripheral sensory polyneuropathy of hands and feet. This was either manifested by changes on objective serial neurological exams measuring vibratory sense or with paresthesias. We were very liberal in calling any neurologic change a drug related neuropathy, despite many of the patients having advancing cancer and worsening nutritional state. The incidence of neurotoxicity is clearly related to total dose, as shown in Table 4, with an overall incidence of 52% in the 93 patients evaluable. Eleven of the 104 patients were not evaluable either because they died after having received only one or two doses of drug or there was not sufficient time for complete evaluation.

TABLE 4

MISONIDAZOLE PHASE I STUDY

Incidence and Grade of Neuropathy as Related to Total Dose in gm/m^2

Total dose gm/m^2	Total incidence of neuropathy	Grade				
		I	II	III	IV	not graded
0-3	0/5	–	–	–	–	–
> 3-6	2/10	1	–	–	–	1
> 6-9	8/17	1	3	2	1	1
> 9-12	13/28	1	5	1	4	2
> 12-15	22/29	2	14	1	5	–
> 15-18	1/2	–	–	–	1	–
> 18-21	2/2	1	1	–	–	–
	48/93 (52%)	6	23	4*	11*	4

*Grade III and IV = 15/93 (16%)

It is not clear that the severity of neuropathy was related to total dose. Table 4 relates the incidence of neuropathy to total dose for the first 93 patients. Most of the neuropathies occurred after the patient approached 10 gm/m^2, usually within one week of that total dose. Whether the incidence of neuropathy, between 3-10 gm/m^2 total dose, is partially related to the advanced tumor state cannot be determined, despite careful neurological screening. At its worst, the neuropathy was associated with weakness and inability to ambulate for up to a period of one week, with progressive weakness and associated changes lasting several weeks thereafter. None of the neuropathies progressed when the drug was stopped; instead the neuropathy improved with time. Patients who had pre-existing neuropathy at the time of entry onto the study did not seem to have a worse neuropathy associated with any given dose. However, patients who had prior vincristine neuropathy clinically developed rapid and severe misonidazole neuropathy, suggesting an additive effect.

Seizures were not observed, except for one patient who had a probable brain metastases from an eye melanoma. Obtundation and mental confusion, encephalopathy, has been observed in several patients and accounts for most of the Grade IV neuropathies. These tended to occur in older patients who became dehydrated, more often debilitated.

The incidence and nature of encephalopathy were further investigated among the Phase I patients. Of 104 patients, 9 were classified as having central nervous system effects typical of encephalopathy. Seven of the 9 were on dose schedules which would have achieved total doses greater than the maximum tolerated doses later established by the Phase I study, i.e., 12 gm/m^2 in 3 weeks or 15 gm/m^2 in

6 weeks. It should be noted, however, that some of the patients did not achieve these totals, since drug was discontinued at the development of encephalopathy. Three of the patients had Grade I encephalopathy with mild confusion and lethargy. Five patients had Grade II encephalopathy with moderate to severe confusion and marked lethargy. One patient had Grade III encephalopathy with reversible coma. No patients had seizures or irreversible coma or death. It is strongly recommended that patients receive adequate hydration throughout their treatment course and that drug be discontinued if adequate hydration cannot be maintained. It is also recommended that drug be discontinued at the first sign of any mental effects.

Ototoxicity, manifested as decreased hearing of a short term duration, was observed in several patients at higher total doses and with dehydration and advanced age.

The development of neuropathy could not be predicted or correlated with any of the pharmacologic parameters of peak sera level, half-life, or percent urinary excretion, but only with total dose administered.

Table 5 shows the acceptable dose schedules of misonidazole, given the dose limiting peripheral neuropathy. The frequency of dose administration has only a mild effect on total doses achievable. Again shown are the blood levels and enhancement ratios expected for key individual drug doses.

TABLE 5

MISONIDAZOLE PHASE I STUDY - ESTABLISHED ACCEPTABLE DOSE SCHEDULES

5-6 gm/m^2	Single dose.
1.5 gm/m^2	Daily X 5-7 days (7.5 - 10.5 gm/m^2).
12 gm/m^2 over 3 weeks }	1-3 divided doses per week
15 gm/m^2 over 6 weeks }	(3-18 doses).

	Serum Level	Enhancement Ratio
1.25 gm/m^2	50 µg/ml	1.5
2.5 gm/m^2	100 µg/ml	1.75

A recent review of our data and data from the W. W. Cross Cancer Institute and the National Cancer Institute (USA)[7] indicates that the incidence of peripheral or central nervous system damage is related to concomitant administration of phenytoin sodium or dexamethasone.

TABLE 6

RELATIONSHIP OF MISONIDAZOLE TOXICITY TO DEXAMETHASONE AND PHENYTOIN INGESTION

Inst.	Dose schedule	± Phenytoin Sodium	± Dexa-methasone	Incidence P.N.	Incidence CNS
UCSF	2 gm/m^2 b.i.w. X 3 wks.	+	+	0/15	0/15
UCSF	2 gm/m^2 b.i.w. X 3 wks.	--	--	4/5	1/5
UCSF	1.25 gm/m^2 b.i.w. X 6 wks.	+	+	0/4	0/4
UCSF	1.25 gm/m^2 b.i.w. X 6 wks.	--	--	6/7	0/7
Cross Ca.Inst.	1.25 gm/m^2 t.i.w. X 3 wks.	--	+	0/9	0/9
Cross Ca.Inst.	1.25 gm/m^2 t.i.w. X 3 wks.	+	+	0/9	0/9
Cross Ca.Inst.	1.25 gm/m^2 t.i.w. X 3 wks.	--	--	5/6	1/6

It is clear that patients receiving similar dose schedules of misonidazole have a much lower incidence of peripheral neuropathy and essentially no incidence of central nervous system injury when given either phenytoin sodium plus dexamethasone or dexamethasone alone. No information is available on patients receiving phenytoin sodium alone. In addition to the apparent protective effect of dexamethasone, it has been observed that phenytoin sodium significantly shortens the half-life (from approximately 11-14 hours to 6-7 hours) following misonidazole administration and seems to increase the excretion of desmethylmisonidazole. There is no evidence that dexamethasone alone shortens the half-life in several patients studied. Both dexamethasone and phenytoin sodium may be useful agents in reducing the incidence of nervous system side effects from misonidazole. Indeed, in the Phase II-III study underway in malignant gliomas in the Brain Tumor Study Group, a very low incidence of peripheral or central neuropathy has been seen in spite of a weekly dose of 3 gm/m^2 and totals ranging from 15-21 gm/m^2. Most of these patients received phenytoin sodium and dexamethasone. On the other hand, doses previously thought tolerable by patients not receiving phenytoin sodium and/or dexamethasone may not be tolerable, and some moderate dosage reductions are planned. The previously established level of 12 gm/m^2 in 3 weeks and 15 gm/m^2 in 6 weeks may be suitable for patients with brain tumors on the above-mentioned agents, but a limit of 10 and 12 gm/m^2, respectively, is needed for patients with other malignancies not taking these agents.

Although the Phase I study was designed to evaluate toxicity and pharmacology, some observations on response of tumors with misonidazole have been obtained. Fifteen patients with malignant glioma were treated with either 400 rads X 12 or 600 rads X 6 with misonidazole given at either 1.25 or 1.5 gm/m^2 with each radiation dose with the 400 rad fractions and at 2 or 2.5 gm/m^2 with the 600 rad fractions. The follow-up to date is incomplete, but suggests that the median survival time, approximately 29 weeks for the 400 rad group and 38 weeks for the patients given 600 rad fractions, is not significantly better than observed previously with radiation alone using conventional fractionation.[8] In addition, several patients are alive at one year following treatment and it may be that long term survival in this group will be better than with conventional radiation although median survival time is not markedly improved.

A number of patients were treated with squamous cell carcinomas of the head and neck region. These all showed excellent to complete responses and it is the clinical impression of the experimenters that the drug is efficacious in these patients. Good responses were seen in carcinomas of the lung and in various histologic type tumors metastatic to the lung and lymph nodes, in particular squamous cell carcinomas. The numbers of patients in other site and histology groups are small. The response of patients with sarcomas and melanomas to large weekly fractions with misonidazole has been disappointing.

Phase II Study

TABLE 7

RTOG PHASE II MISONIDAZOLE STUDIES   (Review 4/15/79)

Study no.	Site	No. pts. entered	Evaluable	*No. periph. nerve toxicity	No. CNS toxicity
78-01	Glioma	32	20	4	0
78-02	H & N weekly	23	13	8	3+
78-12	Brain mets	20	17	0	0
78-13	Hemibody	5	5	0	0∞
78-14	Lung	16	8	1	1
78-15	Sarcoma/ melanoma	8	5	2	0
78-21	Bladder	2	2	1	0
78-23	Recurrent brain	8	1	0	0
78-24	H & N bi-weekly	3	0	0	0
78-30	Liver mets	5	4	1	0
78-31	H & N 3X wkly.	1	0	0	0
	TOTALS:	123	75	17	4

*All Grades--mainly 1, 2.
+2 fatal, 1 Grade-2   (1 fatal possible C.V.A.).
∞1 Grade-2.

In the RTOG Phase II studies, which include gliomas, 3 different head and neck protocols, brain metastases, hemi-body irradiation, lung carcinoma, sarcoma/ melanoma, bladder carcinoma, recurrent brain tumors, liver metastases, and eso- phageal carcinoma, the RTOG has currently accessioned 123 patients as of April 1, 1979 (Table 7). Of 75 evaluable patients, 17 have shown peripheral neuro- pathy and 4 central nervous system toxicity. The majority of these have occur- red in patients with head and neck tumors, necessitating a moderate dose reduc- tion in these patients to a total of 10 gm/m^2 in 3 weeks and 12 gm/m^2 in 6 weeks (Table 8).

TABLE 8

REVISED MISONIDAZOLE DOSES FOR PHASE II STUDIES

Protocol		No. radiation fractions	No. drug doses	Individual Drug Dose	
				Original	Revised
78-01	Glioma	30	6	2.5 gm/m^2	same
78-02	Head and Neck	30	6	2.5 gm/m^2	2.0 gm/m^2
78-12	Brain Metastases	6	6	2.0 gm/m^2	same
79-?		10	6	2.0 gm/m^2	
78-13	Hemibody	1	1	5.0 gm/m^2	4.0 gm/m^2
78-14	Lung	6	6	2.0 gm/m^2	1.75 gm/m^2
79-?		30	10	1.2 gm/m^2	
78-15	Sarcoma/Melanoma	6	6	2.5 gm/m^2	2.0 gm/m^2
78-17	Intra-operative	1	1	3.5 gm/m^2	same
78-21	Bladder	8	8	2.0 gm/m^2	1.5 gm/m^2
78-23	Pediatric Brain	10	6	2.0 gm/m^2	same
78-24	Head and Neck (Marcial)	12	12	1.25 gm/m^2	1.0 gm/m^2
78-30	Liver Metastases	7	7	1.5 gm/m^2	same
78-31	Head and Neck (Order)	11	6	1.75 gm/m^2	1.5 gm/m^2
78-32	Esophagus	12	12	1.25 gm/m^2	1.0 gm/m^2

Following completion of the Phase II studies with 30-40 patients/group and establishment of a tolerable dose schedule, Phase III studies will be activated. It is anticipated that randomized trials for brain metastases and primary car- cinoma of the head and neck will begin in August 1979 in the RTOG.

The RTOG Phase II studies are designed to develop radiation fractionation schemes and drug delivery schemes which will explore 2 major methods of applying the drug. In the first case, conventional fractionation will be coupled with drug delivered once or twice weekly. In this format the radiation is scheduled so that at least 2 of the fractions, and in some cases 4, are accompanied by reasonably high blood levels. This approach is exemplified in the head and neck study, in which 2 fractions are given on the first day of each week in conjunction with a dose of misonidazole and in the planned studies for limited lung cancer and stage IIB and III cervix. In the other approach, a limited number of large fractions is combined with misonidazole at each fraction. This approach is used in the brain metastasis study, the advanced lung carcinoma study, the sarcoma/melanoma study, and in the head and neck pilot studies employing radiation either daily for 11 days or bi-weekly with 400 rad fractions. A limited number of daily fractions each with misonidazole is employed in that head and neck study, in the liver metastasis study, and in the brain metastasis study arm with 300 rads daily for 10 days.

It is hoped through these different approaches that smaller doses of misonidazole given with each fraction can be contrasted with larger doses of misonidazole given less frequently with only a portion of conventional sized fractions. It should be possible to determine whether one gets more enhancement by reducing the number of radiation fractions and using misonidazole with each, or by giving conventional fractionation with misonidazole with only a portion of the fractions.

The only current Phase II-III study in the United States is that of the Brain Tumor Study Group. This study employs conventional radiation fraction to a dose of 6000 rads whole brain with misonidazole given twice weekly. Radiation delivery is scheduled for late one afternoon and early the next morning to take advantage of the prolonged blood levels and tumor levels. To date, toxicity has been acceptable on this regimen. It is too early to compare results with the control arm which utilizes the same fractionation without misonidazole. Both groups received chemotherapy as well.

It is evident that misonidazole has significant neurotoxicity, which precludes its use in sufficiently high doses or with sufficiently large numbers of fractions for optimum sensitization. For this reason the National Cancer Institute of the United States has engaged in a large drug development program for new hypoxic cell sensitizers. This program employs contracts for the synthesis and testing of new analogs, in vitro and in vivo tumor screening of new agents, and clinical trials. The emphasis of the identification and synthesis program is currently on the development of drugs with somewhat shorter half-lives and less lipid solubility in order to attempt to reduce the area under the curve of exposure of the central nervous system, as well as the levels of drug in the

central nervous system. A number of new interesting agents have been synthe-
sized. Several of these have been tested in 3 different mouse tumor models with
3 different endpoints (tumor cure, tumor regrowth delay, and tumor cell survival
analyzed in vitro after in vivo treatment). These tests suggest that some of
the agents are superior to misonidazole, at least as determined by their sensitization as compared to their lethal toxic dose levels. It is planned that the
first of these agents to be studied, Ro-05-9963 (desmethylmisonidazole), a metabolite of misonidazole, will be placed into clinical trial in 1980.

Appropriate dose adjustments with misonidazole and radiation fractionation
schedule adjustments can lead to successful regimens in which the drug can be
used with minimal side effects and in which it appears some sensitization occurs.
We must await the results of randomized clinical trials to determine the extent
to which this drug will be effective in determining the ultimate outcome.

ACKNOWLEDGEMENTS

These studies supported by the National Cancer Institute through the
Radiation Therapy Oncology Group (Grant No. CA-21439). Misonidazole supplied
by the Drug Development Branch, Division of Cancer Treatment, National Cancer
Institute.

REFERENCES

1. Denekamp, J. (1978) Int. J. Radiat. Oncology Biol. Phys., 4, 143-151.

2. Dische, S. (1978) Int. J. Radiat. Oncology Biol. Phys., 4, 157-160.

3. Wasserman, T. H., et al. (1979) Int. J. Radiat. Oncology Biol. Phys.,
   (in press).

4. McNally, N. J., et al. (1978) Radiat. Res., 73, 568-580.

5. Dische, S., et al. (1976) Clin. Radiol., 27, 159-167.

6. Johnson, R., et al. (1976) Int. J. Radiat. Oncology Biol. Phys., 1, 593-599.

7. Wasserman, T. H., et al. (in press) Brit. J. Radiol., Letter to the Editor
   on Neurotoxicity of Misonidazole: Potential Modifying Role of Phenytoin
   Sodium and Dexamethasone.

8. Wara, W. M., et al. (1980) Int. J. Radiat. Oncology Biol. Phys.,
   (in press).

HYPERTHERMIA

© 1979, Elsevier/North-Holland Biomedical Press
Treatment of Radioresistant Cancers
M. Abe, K. Sakamoto and T.L. Phillips eds.

EFFECT OF FRACTIONATED HYPERTHERMIA ON NORMAL AND TUMOR TISSUES IN AN EXPERIMENTAL ANIMAL SYSTEM[**]

MUNEYASU URANO[*], LAURIE RICE AND MARY CUNNINGHAM
Department of Radiation Medicine, Massachusetts General Hospital and Harvard
Medical School, Boston, Massachusetts 02114, U.S.A.

INTRODUCTION

Biological features of the radioresistant tumors may vary from one tumor to another. Tumor cells may be intrinsically resistant to ionizing radiation. The cells may possess a greater capability of repairing sublethal and/or potentially lethal radiation damage. Tumor cells surviving after doses may still be capable of proliferating rapidly with an increased growth fraction and/or decreased cell loss factor. The tumor may contain a large fraction of radioresistant tumor cells, i.e., a large fraction of cells in S phase or clonogenic hypoxic tumor cells. The tumor may be resistant because of unsuccessful reoxygenation occurring during a fractionated radiotherapy. Besides this true resistance, the apparent resistant tumor may be due to slow regression.

Many attempts have been made to achieve better tumor control rate compared to conventional radiotherapy, including the use of hyperbaric oxygen, radiosensitizers, high LET radiations, altered fractionation regimen, combined use of chemotherapy, etc. None of these attempts have been reported to be fully successful.

Hyperthermia may be a potential source of cancer treatment[1,2]. Recent studies have revealed its biological effectiveness on mammalian cells[3,4]. Heat treatment at moderate temperature can lethally damage mammalian cells. The treatment time vs. cell survival relation, like radiation dose - cell survival relations, exhibits an exponential relation which follows an initial shoulder. Rationale for use of hyperthermia in the treatment of radioresistant tumors might be that (a) hypoxic cells are at least as sensitive as aerobic cells to hyperthermia[5-9], (b) the S-phase cells which are resistant to ionizing radiation in most cell lines are more sensitive to heat as compared to G_1 cells[10,11] and (c) hyperthermia induces an extensive division delay (or inhibits cell progression extensively) relative to radiations[12]. This presentation will be

---

[**]Supported in part by NCI Grant #CA13311, D.H.E.W.
[*]To whom requests for reprints should be addressed.

restricted to hyperthermia-alone treatment with a limited attention to combined heat and radiation therapy, which may offer numerous attractive features for treatment of radioresistant tumors.

We have attempted without success to cure some spontaneous murine tumors with a tolerable single level of hyperthermia. Tumors growing in the mouse foot pad were treated at 43.5°C in a hot waterbath. Tumor control was found to be associated with a severe foot reaction, namely, loss of at least one toe or occasionally loss of foot. TCD_{50} (treatment time required to achieve local tumor control in half the treated animals) was found for most of the tumors to be greater than RD_{50} (≥ 4.0)[*], i.e., treatment time which produces loss of one toe or greater foot reaction in half the treated animals (Table 1). For example, RD_{50} of our animals was 140 min while TCD_{50}s of spontaneous mouse fibrosarcoma (FSa-II) and mammary carcinoma were 170 and ≈140 min, respectively. Hepatoma was controlled only in animals with foot amputated. In the same table, TCD_{50}s by single radiation dose for these tumors obtained in our laboratory are also listed[13-15]. It is of interest to note that the thermal sensitivity of tumors is proportioned to their radiation sensitivity. In other words, radioresistant tumors also appeared to be heat-resistant. These results emphasize the necessity of different approaches to heat treatment. One such approach is unquestionably the search for a satisfactory fractionation regimen.

TABLE 1

TCD_{50} VALUES OF VARIOUS MURINE TUMORS IN C3H/SED MICE

FSa-I is a methylcholanthrene-induced fibrosarcoma while all others are early generation isotransplants of spontaneous tumors. Tumor size at the time of hyperthermia or irradiation was 4 mm or 8 mm in average diameter respectively except FSa-I which received heat treatment at 6 mm.

Tumor	TCD_{50} (Heat) (min)	TCD_{50} (Radiat)[*] (rad)
FSa-I[**]	78	3400
Mammary ca.	≈140	6550
FSa-II	170	7805
Sq. cell ca.	≈195	8020
Hepatoma	>200	8500
RD_{50} (≥ 5.0)	180	–
RD_{50} (≥ 4.0)	140	–

*Suit, H.D. et al.   **Chemically-induced

[*] will be abbreviated RD_{50}

EXPERIMENTAL MATERIALS AND METHODS

Animals were 10-12 week old C3Hf/Sed mice derived from our specific pathogen-free and defined flora colony[16]. They were kept in our animal facility where defined flora conditions have been maintained. Sterilized Wayne Lab Blox and acidified and vitamin K-fortified water were provided ad libitum. Experimental tumors were 8th generation isotransplants of a mouse fibrosarcoma which arose spontaneously in a female C3Hf/Sed mouse. This tumor was designated FSa-II. A single cell suspension was prepared by trypsinization[17] and approximately 2 to 5 x 10^5 viable tumor cells in 5 μℓ was transplanted into the right foot. The tumor volume doubling time at 100-200 mm^3 was approximately 2 days. This tumor was weakly immunogenic[18].

Localized hyperthermia was given by immersing mouse feet in a hot waterbath maintained at 43.5 ± 0.05°C by a constant temperature circulator (Haake Model E52). Tissue temperature was no less than 43.4°C. No anesthesia was administered during treatment.

The tumor response was studied by TG (Tumor Growth) time analysis[19]. Animals were randomly assigned into groups after transplantation. Hyperthermia was given when tumors reached 6 mm average diameter. After treatment, three diameters of each tumor were measured at least 4 times a week. The tumor volume was calculated as an elipsoid and then plotted as a function of time after treatment. The TG time from treatment day until the tumors reached 1000 mm^3 was obtained graphically in each tumor and the median TG time required for half the treated tumors to reach 1000 mm^3 was calculated by logit analysis. In each dose group, 6 to 10 animals were used.

Normal tissue response was studied by scoring the foot reaction. Animals were randomized into groups and then the right feet were treated. Foot reaction was scored according to a numerical scoring system (Table 2) between day 6 and 35 after treatment; every day during 1st week with decreasing frequency in subsequent days, and the average peak foot reaction was obtained in each group. The scoring was performed by an examiner who has no prior knowledge of the identity of animals. It must be mentioned that this numerical score system includes 2 different types of reactions; reversible skin reaction and irreversible bone damage. The same data was also used for calculation of RD_{50}. In an RD_{50} assay, 30 to 50 animals were used with 5 to 10 mice in each dose group.

TABLE 2

NUMERICAL SCORE SYSTEM OF THE MOUSE FOOT REACTION AFTER HYPERTHERMIA

Scores 0-3.5 represent reversible skin reaction while scores greater than 4.0 are due to irreversible damage.

0   : Normal foot

0.5: 50% Chance of damage

1.0: Red foot, partial epilation

1.5: Slight edema, epilation

2.0: Severe edema, complete epilation

2.5: Fusion of toes

3.0: Partial wet desquamation

3.5: Wet desquamation of most of foot

4.0: Loss of 1 toe, (Loss of 1 to 4 segments)

4.5: Loss of more than 2 toes (More than 5 segments)

5.0: Loss of foot

6.0: Loss of leg up to the ankle

RESULTS AND DISCUSSION

Split Dose Effect. Mammalian cells surviving the 1st heat treatment have been reported to become resistant to subsequent treatments. This heat resistance develops in the first 2 days and is then gradually lost over several days[20-22]. This phenomenon was also observed in animal tissue as presented in Figure 1. Animal feet received 2 equal doses with various time intervals between treatments (Ti) and RD_{50} was determined. An increase of RD_{50} can be seen in the figure with increasing time up to 48 hours and is followed by gradual decrease. In addition to the development and loss of heat resistance, it is notable as seen in Figure 1 that, first, the split dose RD_{50} was always greater than single dose RD_{50} even after the heat resistance was lost; secondly, the RD_{50} with Ti of 10 days was no greater than RD_{50} with Ti of 5 days. The former phenomenon might indicate that the normal tissue cells were able to repair sublethal or potentially lethal heat damage or that the heat resistance was never fully lost. The second might suggest no increase of surviving tissue cells in this 5 days or continuous decrease of heat sensitivity with or without proliferation of surviving tissue cells.

RD_{50} vs. Overall Treatment Time. The development and the loss of heat resistance, as well as possible repair capability of surviving cells, may form a unique feature in fractionated hyperthermia. Two types of fractionation regimens were studied, namely, Ti of 2 and 5 days. These Ti's were chosen since heat resistance fully develops in 2 days and is lost to insignificant level in 5 days. Animal feet were treated with multiple equal doses and RD_{50} (≥ 4.0) was analyzed. As shown in Figure 2, RD_{50} (≥ 4.0) increased with increasing overall treatment time (or increasing number of fractions). This increase was substantial for Ti of 2 days as compared to that for Ti of 5 days. A linear regression line can be fitted between RD_{50} and overall treatment time (or number of fractions) for each regimen, although the relation for Ti of 2 days has a breaking point when the overall treatment time exceeds 2 days, i.e., the development of heat resistance might be less extensive after 2nd heat treatment.

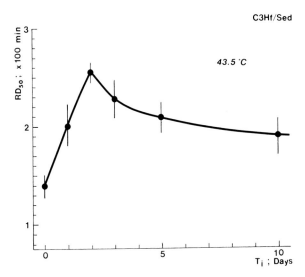

Fig. 1. Effect of split doses on RD_{50} (≥ 4.0) in C3Hf/Sed mice. Two equal doses were given with various time intervals (Ti) and the RD_{50} (≥ 4.0), i.e., the treatment time to induce "loss of a toe" or more severe reaction, was determined at 35 days after treatment. Vertical bars indicate 95% confidence limit.

Average Peak Foot Reaction After Multiple Doses. Some of the above data were further analyzed. The average peak foot reaction in each dose group was plotted as a function of total dose (Figure 3). The relation between the treatment time and average score appeared to be an exponential relation rather than a linear one. It is of interest to note that the slopes for multiple fractions were more steep than that for single treatment. This suggests more extensive recovery of surviving tissue cells after small doses relative to after large doses. The ratio of treatment time to induce average peak score

48

5.0 or 1.0 (i.e., a large or small dose) after 6 doses with Ti of 2 days to that after single dose was 3.3 or 5.3 respectively. No definite interpretation can be made for the large recovery observed at shorter treatment time, although several hypotheses are available. An attractive hypothesis might be that a large heat dose gave severe tissue damage with the decrease of tissue pH which increased thermal response of the tissue cells[4,7,23,24] or markedly inhibited repopulation of surviving cells.

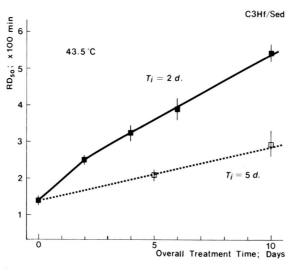

Fig. 2. Time-dose relationship for RD_{50} (≥4.0). Multiple treatments were given with Ti of 2 days (solid squares) or 5 days (open squares), and RD_{50}s (≥4.0) in 35 days are plotted as a function of overall treatment days. Vertical bars indicate 95% confidence limit.

TG Time After Multiple Doses. The same treatment regimen, i.e., Ti of 2 and 5 days, used for normal tissue response was also studied for tumor response. Tumors in foot pad received multi-treatments and the TG time was analyzed. An exponential relation was observed between TG time and treatment time at 43.5°C for all the fractionation regimens (Figure 4). The dose response curves for Ti of 2 days were less steep than those for single dose, indicating that the heat sensitivity to the 2nd dose decreased dramatically in 2 days; namely, the tumor cells became heat-resistant. This phenomenon was obvious for 6 doses as compared to 2 doses and indicates heat resistance is not lost in the fractionated treatments with Ti of 2 days. Unlike the normal tissue response, the ratio of treatment time to induce a given TG time by multi-treatments to that by single dose appeared to be independent of fraction size. The ratio of treatment time to induce the TG time of 10 or 20 days by 6 doses was 3.4 or

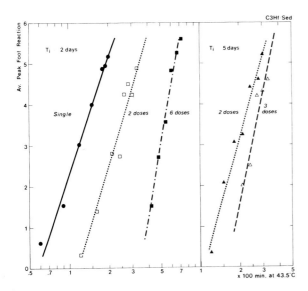

Fig. 3. Dose response curves for average peak foot reaction. Left panel includes treatments with Ti of 2 days together with single treatment while the right panel is for treatment with a Ti of 5 days. Standard deviations are omitted for clarity.

3.5 respectively. On the contrary, the dose response curves for Ti of 5 days was shifted to the right with no appreciable changes in the slope. Presumably, tumor cells were able to repair sublethal heat damage in 5 days with loss of heat resistance. Possible repopulation of surviving tumor cells may partially contribute to shift the curve to the right. A difference between the treatment time to achieve a given TG time by multidoses with Ti of 5 days and that by single dose increases with increasing number of fractions. It was approximately 20 and 55 min for 2 and 3 doses, indicating that the tumor cells were capable of repairing sublethal damage repeatedly after each dose.

  Differential Response. The relationship between TG time and average peak foot reaction can be derived from dose response curves of normal and tumor tissues shown in Figures 3 and 4[*]. At any level of foot reactions, the prolongation of TG time was obvious for any fractionation regimen tested (Figure

---

[*]Relationship between the average score of foot reaction (FR) and the treatment time (T), and that between the TG time (TGT) and T are;

$$FR = a \log T + b$$
$$\log TGT = c \, T + d$$

Hence, $\log \log TGT = A \cdot FR + B$

where a, b, c, d, A and B are constant.

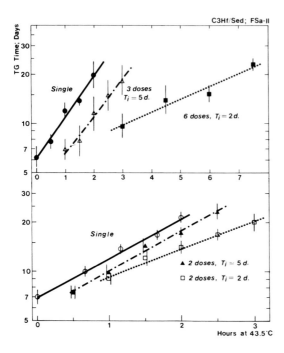

Fig. 4. Dose response curves for TG time of FSa-II tumors transplanted into foot pad. First, treatment was given when tumors reached 6 mm in average diameter. TG time, i.e., the time required for half the treated tumors to reach 1000 mm^3 from first treatment day, was plotted as a function of total treatment time. Multiple treatments were given in equal doses. The top figure indicates the treatments with an overall treatment time of 10 days and the bottom figure shows treatments with 2 equal doses. Vertical bars are 95% confidence limit.

5). For Ti of 2 days, the prolongation was more appreciable at short treatment time and decreased with increasing treatment time to an insignificant level. Accordingly, the preferable differential response could be obtained only by a relatively short, i.e., non-curable, treatment time. For Ti of 5 days, however, the prolongation was uniformly observed throughout all levels of foot reaction, indicating that the differential response is likely by any fraction size.

CONCLUSION

Figure 6 compares time-dose relationships of normal and tumor tissues. Doses are plotted as a ratio of total dose to single dose which yields a given level of tissue response. Foot and tumor responses are RD$_{50}$ and treatment time to produce TG time of 20 days respectively. These data are taken from Figures 2 and 4. The total dose to give rise to such reactions increases with

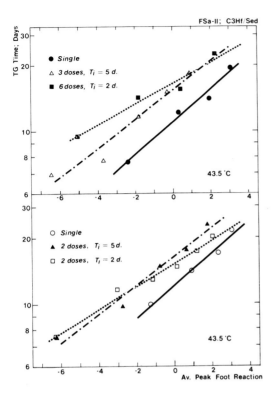

Fig. 5. Relationship between TG time and average peak foot reaction. Data shown in Figures 2 and 4 are used. Negative values in foot reaction were due to regression analysis of the dose response curves for foot reaction (see previous footnote). Top figure includes treatments with overall treatment time of 10 days and the bottom indicates 2 equal doses.

increasing overall treatment time. For Ti of 2 days, this increase in tumor response dose was comparable to that in RD_{50}, indicating insignificant development of differential responses with increasing overall time. It must be mentioned, however, that the treatments of heat-sensitive tumors with a Ti of 2 days may result in preferable differential response as shown in Figure 5. The treatments of heat-sensitive FSa-I with a Ti of ≃1 day are reported to improve the therapeutic ratio[25]. Interestingly, for Ti of 5 days, the increase in the tumor response dose was less pronounced than that in RD_{50}. It is very likely that the preferable differential response becomes more appreciable with increasing overall time or increasing number of fractions. A possible explanation for the less pronounced increase is; tumor cells were less capable of repairing sublethal damage as compared to normal tissue cells, or thermal

52

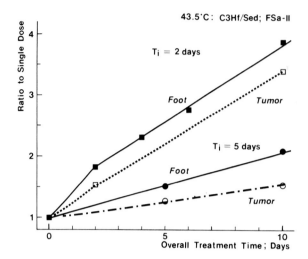

Fig. 6. Comparison of the time-dose relationship for foot reaction and that for tumor response. Ratio of total dose to single dose to yield a given level of reaction was plotted instead of total doses for simple presentation. The foot reaction was RD_{50} (≥ 4.0) taken from Figure 2 and the tumor response was the treatment time to yield TG time of 20 days which was obtained from Figure 4. The top two and bottom two curves are treatments with Ti of 2 days and those with Ti of 5 days respectively. Open and solid symbols indicate tumor and foot reaction respectively.

sensitivity of tumor cells may be enhanced during the fractionated treatments. Presumably heat damage in the blood vessels may be associated with decreased tissue pH which makes tumor cells sensitive to subsequent treatments[4,7;23,24]. Whatever the mechanism is, present results indicate that with the appropriate fractionation regimen, hyperthermia alone might be a potential treatment method of the radioresistant tumor.

ACKNOWLEDGEMENT

We acknowledge Drs. H.D. Suit and L.E. Gerweck for their valuable discussions and supports throughout these studies.

REFERENCES

1. Miller, R.C. et. al. (1977) Radiology 123, 489-495,

2. Suit, H.D. and Schwayder, M. (1974) Cancer 34, 122-129.

3. Dewey, W.C. et. al. (1977) Radiology 123, 463-474.

4. Gerweck, L.E. (1977) Radiat. Res. 70, 224-235.

5. Gerweck, L.E. et al. (1974) Europ. J. Cancer 10, 691-693.

6. Gerweck, L.E. et. al. (1979) Cancer Res. 39, 966-972.

7. Overgaard, J. and Bichel, P. (1977) Radiology 123, 511-514.

8. Power, J.A. and Harris, J.W. (1977) Radiology 123, 767-770.

9. Robinson, J.E. (1975) Proceedings of the International Symposium on Cancer Therapy by Hyperthermia and Radiation, April 28-30, Washington, D.C.

10. Westra, A. and Dewey, W.C. (1971) Int. J. Radiat. Biol. 19, 467-477.

11. Lucke-Huhle, C. and Dertinger, H. (1977) Europ. J. Cancer 13, 23-28.

12. Sapareto, S.A. et. al. (1978) Cancer Res. 38, 393-400.

13. Suit, H.D. and Brown, J.M. (1979) Brit. J. Radiology 52, 159-160.

14. Suit, H.D. and Maimonis, P. Personal Communication.

15. Suit, H.D. et. al. (1976) Cancer Res. 36, 1305-1314.

16. Sedlacek, R.S. and Mason, K.A. (1977) Laboratory Animal Sci. 27, 667-670.

17. Urano, M. et. al. (1976) Radiology 118, 447-451.

18. Urano, M. et. al. (In Press). Cancer Res.

19. Urano, M. et. al. (1974) J. Natl. Cancer Inst. 53, 517-525.

20. Gerner, E.W. et. al. (1976) Cancer Res. 36, 1035-1040.

21. Harisiadis, L. et. al. (1977) Radiology 123, 505-509.

22. Henle, K.J. and Dethlefsen, L.A. (1978) Cancer Res. 38, 1843-1851.

23. Freeman, M.L. et. al. (1977) J. Natl. Cancer Inst. 58, 1837-1839.

24. von Ardenne, M. and Reitnauer, P.G. (1978) J. Natl. Cancer Inst. 61, 3-4.

25. Suit, H.D. (1977) Radiology 123, 483-487.

© 1979, Elsevier/North-Holland Biomedical Press
Treatment of Radioresistant Cancers
M. Abe, K. Sakamoto and T.L. Phillips eds.

CELL KILLING BY HYPERTHERMIA AND RADIATION IN CANCER THERAPY.

CHRISTIAN STREFFER, DIRK VAN BEUNINGEN and NIKOLAUS ZAMBOGLOU
Institut für Med. Strahlenphysik und Strahlenbiologie, Universitätsklinikum Essen, Hufelandstr. 55, 43 Essen 1 (W.-Germany)

INTRODUCTION

Cell killing is an essential event for tumor therapy. If we consider cell killing by ionizing radiation in tumors we are faced with two major problems:

1) In tumors there are regions with hypoxic cells which are relatively radioresistant against ionizing radiation with low LET.

2) Cell populations may occur in the tumor with a high capacity for recovery, for which the survival is relatively large in the dose range of 100-400 Rads.

Combined modalities will be especially effective if they can affect these cell populations. For the decision on the usefulness of hyperthermia in tumor therapy it is therefore of special interest whether hyperthermia can alter and enhance the radiation effects on such cells.

INFLUENCE OF HYPOXIA AND METABOLISM

Recently a number of authors have shown that hypoxic cells exhibit greater sensitivity to hyperthermia than well oxygenated cells[1]. The extent of this effect is considerably higher after mammalian cells have been cultivated under hypoxic conditions for a longer period than after acute hypoxia[2,3]. Gerweck et al.[3] have studied the survival of Chinese hamster ovary (CHO) cells after hypoxia and irradiation. Sensitivity to hyperthermia increases when the time of culture under hypoxia is longer. In contrast the cells are protected against irradiation by hypoxia even when the cells are cultured under hypoxic conditions for 30 hours.

Apparently metabolic changes have occurred in these cells which lead for instance to a lowering of the pH-value and thus to a sensitization of the cells against heat[3]. Such an effect has been proposed very strongly by v. Ardenne[4]. Also it has been demonstrated by several authors[3,4] that the pH-value in the interstitial fluid is lower in tumors than in normal tissues like muscle and liver. This difference can be enhanced by glucose infusion and also by hyperthermia[4]. It has been discussed that the acidification of tissues by hyperthermia is caused through an increase of lactate levels. However metabolic studies in mouse liver show that the strongly acidic metabolites β-hydroxybutyrate and acetoacetate are tremendously enhanced after whole body hyperthermia, while lactate is even decreased[5].

It must be assumed that these and other metabolic changes and not the alteration of the H^+-concentration per se are of great importance and are significant for the higher heat sensitivity of mammalian cells. From such metabolic studies more explanation of the mechanism may be obtained.

The described metabolic changes after prolonged hypoxia and after hyperthermia together increase the sensitivity of cells against hyperthermia. Such effects are apparently more prominent in tumors than in normal tissues. Under such circumstances a hyperthermia treatment will be favorable in order to kill hypoxic cells in tumors.

ACTION ON RECOVERY PROCESSES AND CELL KILLING

If one considers the second aspect - namely relatively radioresistent cells with a high recovery capacity - it has frequently been shown that hyperthermia interferes with repair processes[1,6]. Clark and Lett[6] found a decreased repair of radiation damage through the inhibition of the repair of single strand breaks after hyperthermia. The effect was dependent on the temperature. These data are consistent with the observation that those cells with a high recovery which are more radioresistant are comparatively sensitive to heat. Investigations with synchronized cells have resulted in a high heatsensitivity for cells in late S-phase where the survival after irradiation has been highest[7,8]. The survival curves of these cells in late S-phase show a broad shoulder after irradiation without hyperthermia which is taken as a strong evidence for recovery processes.

We have studied the combined effects of hyperthermia and irradiation of a human melanoma cell line with a relatively broad shoulder in the survival curve ($D_q \sim 250$ R) when the colony forming ability is tested[9]. The plating efficiency of this established cell line is about 80 percent. The asynchronously growing cells have been cultivated in Minimum Essential Medium with 15 percent calf serum and addition of 1 percent amino acid and 1 mM Na-pyruvate. The medium has been buffered with $NaHCO_3/CO_2$ at pH 7.4. Per culture $5 \cdot 10^5$ cells have been incubated in 5 ml medium usually at 37° C.

The cells grow for 96 hours in an exponential way and then level off almost into a plateau phase (Fig. 1). Figure 1 represents the average DNA content per culture plotted in a logarithmic scale against incubation time. The DNA content has been determined with a slightly modified method according to Burton[9]. It has been shown by cell counting that these measurements are proportional to the cell number.

In further experiments the melanoma cells have been incubated at various temperatures for 3 hours. This treatment has always been started 24 hours after the cells have been brought into the culture medium. The incubation at 40° C has no effect on the cell growth. After treatment at 42° C a small delay is observed and the cells reach a smaller plateau. The effects are strongly enhanced when the cells are incubated at 44° C. Under these conditions even a decrease of the DNA content per culture occurs at the longer incubation periods (Fig. 1). These data demonstrate that the treatment of the cells at 44° C has a strong cytotoxic effect.

As already stated small X-ray doses up to 200 R have more or less no effect on the cell growth[9]. Also an irradiation with 400 R reduces the increase of the DNA content in comparison to the untreated cultures only to a slight degree. This observation demonstrates again the relatively high radioresistance of these melanoma cells. However, when the melanoma cells have been incubated for 3 hours at 42° C after an X-ray dose of 400 R the cell growth is strongly affected (Fig. 2). After a delay of some hours the DNA content rises with about the same rate for 48 hours. After this period the DNA content decreases rapidly which is

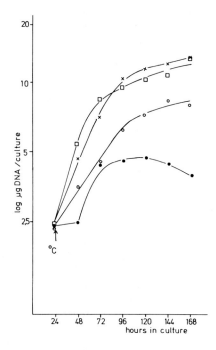

Fig. 1   DNA content per culture of human melanoma
cells after hyperthermia x——x controls;
□——□ 3 hours at 40° C; o——o 3 hours at 42° C;
●——● 3 hours at 44° C.

apparently due to cell loss. At these later periods a large
number of cells has been found unattached to the bottom of the
flask in the culture medium. This has been in contrast to the
untreated cultures. The cells in the medium are classified as
dead cells, they are stained by trypan blue.

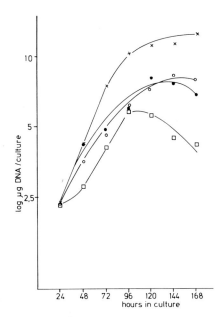

Fig. 2   DNA content per culture of human
melanoma cells after hyperthermia and irradiation
x——x controls; o——o 3 hours at 42° C;
●——● 400 R X-rays; □——□ 400 R X-rays plus
3 hours at 42° C.

These results are a good evidence for a strong synergistic
effect of the combination of irradiation and hyperthermia on cell
killing. The synergism is most pronounced at moderate temperatures as 40° C and 42° C which may be important for the clinical
application, as the elevation of the tissue temperature to such a
degree can be accomplished more easily (Fig. 3).

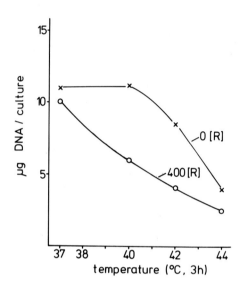

Fig. 3   DNA content per culture of human
melanoma cells 144 hours after hyperthermia
alone x——x and after hyperthermia plus
400 R X-rays o——o

    Little synergistic effect is seen at the cytotoxic temperature
of 44° C. Furthermore Figure 3 shows the steep gradient between
40° and 44° C. For clinical use this phenomenon within the small
dose range must be cautiously observed.

DNA SYNTHESIS AND PROLIFERATION OF MELANOMA CELLS
    Further studies have been performed in order to explorate the
mechanism of the combined modality. For that reason the DNA
synthesis and especially the proliferation kinetics of the melano-

ma cells have been investigated. In order to measure the rate of
DNA synthesis the culture medium has been removed. After trypsinization the cells have been incubated with fresh culture medium and
^{3}H-thymidine (1 μCi/ml; specif. activity 48 Ci/mmole) for
7.5-15 minutes. The DNA has been isolated by a biochemical method
and the incorporated radioactivity has been measured in a liquid
scintillation counter[9]. The rate of ^{3}H-thymidine incorporation
was linear over the mentioned period.

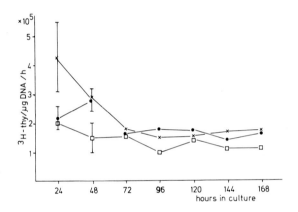

Fig. 4   DNA synthesis rate of human melanoma cells expressed
as ^{3}H-thymidine incorporation per μg DNA per hour. x——x controls;
●——● 3 hours at 42° C; □——□ 400 R X-rays plus 3 hours at 42° C.

If the incorporated radioactivity is calculated on the basis
of the DNA content per culture (dpm/μg DNA/hour), this value
decreases with the culturing time, reaches a plateau at about
72 hours and stays at this plateau for the further period
(Fig. 4). The reason for such a shape of the curve is unclear
up to now. The possibility exists that the intracellular,
endogenous pool of thymidine may change which will influence the
incorporation rate of ^{3}H-thymidine into the DNA. However, by the use
of different specific activities for the ^{3}H-thymidine the same

kind of curve has been obtained. Thus the observed phenomenon has
to be clarified.

Irradiation of the melanoma cells with 400 R has only minor
effects on the rate of DNA synthesis. Directly after the cells
have been incubated at 42° C for three hours the rate of DNA
synthesis is reduced in the melanoma cells, the normal value is
reached some hours later. However, the combination of irradiation
and hyperthermia causes a decreased rate of DNA synthesis over a
longer time. At the later periods the ^{3}H-thymidine incorporation
into the DNA has been unchanged after all treatment conditions.
This is especially surprising for the combined modality. Despite
the enormous cell loss at the later incubation periods the
remaining cells, which are still attached to the culture flask,
synthesize DNA at the same rate as untreated cells (Fig. 4).
The strong depression of the DNA synthesis, which has been
observed directly after the treatment, may contribute to the
observed growth delay.

For such an explanation the determination of the proliferation
kinetics will be of great value. Cell nuclei of the melanoma cells
have been prepared. The cell nuclei are stained with ethidiumbromide after fixation on a slide by incubation with $7.5 \cdot 10^{-5}$ M
ethidiumbromide in 0.1 M phosphate buffer pH 7.5 for 90 minutes
in the dark. The fluorescence has been measured at a wavelength
of 580 nm (excitation 490 nm) with a microscope photometer
MPV 2 (Leitz, Wetzlar)[9]. The same nuclei have also been used
for autoradiography after incubation with ^{3}H-thymidine as
described before. The cell nuclei have been dipped in Ilford K2
photoemulsion and exposed for two weeks. By these two techniques
it is possible to determine the distribution of the cells in the
cell cycle, the labelling index and also to decide for each
individual cell whether it is labelled after having measured its
DNA content.

When the percentage of cells in S-phase has been measured and
compared with the labelling index, a good agreement is seen for
both parameters in untreated melanoma cells (Fig. 5). In contrast to this observation the relative number of cells in S-phase
decreased when the melanoma cells have been irradiated with 400 R
and incubated for 3 hours at 42° C. However the reduction of the

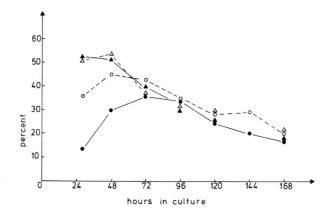

Fig. 5   Percentage of cells in S-phase (▲,●) and labelling
index (Δ,o) of human melanoma cells. (▲,Δ) controls;
(●,o) 400 R X-rays plus 3 hours at 42° C.

labelling index has been much less than the depression of the
S-phase cells (Fig. 5). This can only be explained on the basis
that not only cells in S-phase are labelled but also cells in
other phases of the cell cycle.

Such cells are mainly found in the G_1-phase. In untreated
melanoma cells only about 5 percent of the G_1-phase cells have
been labelled. This effects is mainly due to technical reasons,
as the reproducibility of the DNA determination (Fig. 6). In
contrast to this situation about 35 percent of the G_1-phase cells
are labelled directly after the combined treatment and this
situation is continuing for about 24 hours. After that period
again only a very small number of cells in G_1-phase is labelled
(Fig. 6).

These data further demonstrate that it is not possible to conclude how many cells are in S-phase from the labelling index
alone after a serious treatment. It has to be discussed whether
the label in the G_1-phase cells is due to unscheduled DNA

64

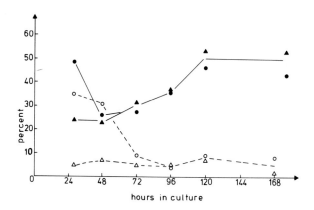

Fig. 6   Percentage of cells in G_1-phase (▲,●) and
of labelled G_1-phase (Δ,o) of human melanoma cells.
(▲,Δ) controls; (●,o) 400 R X-rays plus 3 hours
at 42° C.

synthesis. Such a possibility is supported by preliminary data
which have been obtained by experiments with hydroxyurea. When
the cells are incubated with ^{3}H-thymidine plus hydroxyurea after
the combined treatment it is found that the labelling index is
depressed in the S-phase cells where semiconservative and possibly
unscheduled DNA synthesis may occur and it is unchanged in G_1-
phase cells where only unscheduled DNA synthesis can happen.

If one looks for the distribution of cells in the cell cycle
without further treatment, it is observed, that with continuing
incubation the number of G_1-phase cells increases from around
25 percent to more than 50 percent while the number of S-phase
cells decreases. The number of cells in S-phase is reduced
3 hours after X-irradiation with 400 R (27 hours "old", Fig. 7).
At the same time the number of cells in G_1-phase is somewhat
increased.

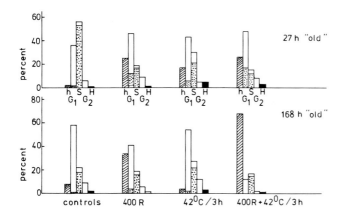

Fig. 7   Distribution of human melanoma cells in the cell cycle
and labelled cells [:::] in the different cell cycle phases
h: hypoploid cells; H: hyperploid cells.

FORMATION OF HYPOPLOID CELLS AND MICRONUCLEI

After irradiation alone and especially after the combined
treatment of X-rays plus hyperthermia a new class of cell nuclei
appears. These are cell nuclei which show a DNA content lower
than that of a diploid genome. We call these cells hypoploid cells.
During the incubation period the number of these cells increases
after irradiation alone and to a much higher degree after the
combined treatment. Concomittant with this development less cells
are found in G_1-phase. There occur also some cell nuclei with a
DNA content which is higher than that of the G_2-phase cells
(hyperploid cells), but the number is small (Fig. 7). The
number of cells in G_2-phase does not change considerably under
all investigated situations. When the DNA content has been
measured in those cells which are no longer attached to the
culture flask and which appear in the medium, it is found that
most of the cells have a DNA content which is characteristic for
hypoploid cell. These cells are stained by trypan blue.

Such effects have been observed only to a small extent after
treatment with hyperthermia alone, even when the incubation
temperature is raised to 44° C. Directly after incubation at 42° C
for 3 hours some hypoploid cells also appear after heating alone,
but during the following incubation period these cells are
apparently detached from the bottom of the culture flask. At later
periods the hypoploid cells are not observed to a higher extent
after hyperthermia alone (Fig. 7). Only when the more cytotoxic
temperature of 44° C is used, some increase of the number of
hypoploid cells occurs, but again not to that degree which is
found after a comparable X-ray dose and combined treatment
(unpublished data).

The hypoploid cells are apparently formed through a release of
chromatin from the cell nuclei. If the cell nuclei from untreated
cells are observed under the microscope after staining with
ethidiumbromide, they appear very nicely round shaped. Such well
formed cell nuclei are not seen after the combined treatment.
Aside these cell nuclei small pieces of stained material, probably
chromatin, can be found. These released chromatin pieces are
called micronuclei (Fig. 8). The occurrence of the micronuclei
is considered as a sign for cytogenetic damage[10], it is equivalent to chromosome breakage.

The number of micronuclei has been determined in relation to
the number of cells (Fig. 9). In untreated cells very few
micronuclei are seen, after incubation at 42° C for 3 hours only
a relatively small increase of this phenomenon occurs. This
effect is higher after X-irradiation alone and is maximal after
the combined treatment. The difference is most pronounced after
a period of 72 hours in culture. It is proposed that the development of these events contribute to cell killing after irradiation
and after the combined modality. However, the cytotoxic effect of
hyperthermia alone may be caused by other processes. Even the
incubation for 3 hours at 44° C, a cytotoxic exposure, causes
only a small increase in the number of micronuclei.

This would mean that the mechanism for the cytotoxic effect by
heat alone is quite different from that for the radiosensitizing
effect of hyperthermia. Our data are in good agreement with
results obtained by Dewey and Sapareto[11] who have found a cor-

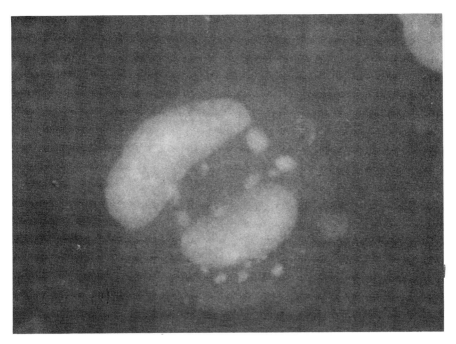

Fig. 8   Cell nuclei of human melanoma cells and formation
of micronuclei stained by ethidiumbromide. 400 x

relation between the occurrence of chromosome aberrations and
cell killing after X-irradiation alone and after X-irradiation
plus hyperthermia. Radiosensitization by hyperthermia apparently
occurs by enhancing radiation induced damage at the chromatin
level or at least in the cell nucleus. As the "hyperthermia dose"
alone which has been used in these experiments, has been moderate
and only causes little nuclear changes of the investigated type,
it is very probable that in the combined treatment the incubation
at elevated temperatures interferes with repair processes after
irradiation.

Several authors have described that hyperthermic exposures can
induce a transient resistance to subsequent heat exposures[12-14].
Such a phenomenon, which has been called thermotolerance, is very

68

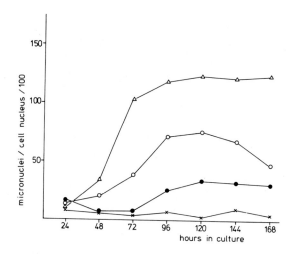

Fig. 9   Formation of micronuclei of human melanoma
cells expressed as micronuclei per cell nucleus x 100.
x——x controls; ●——● 3 hours at 42° C; o——o 400 R X-rays;
Δ——Δ 400 R X-rays plus 3 hours at 42° C.

important for fractionated treatments and therefore significant
for the clinical application of hyperthermia. It has to be eluci-
dated whether such phenomena also occur during repeated combined
treatment. First experiments show that thermotolerance is small
or even not seen at all when the fractionated heating is combined
with irradiation.

CONCLUSIONS

A number of biological investigations have demonstrated that
hypoxic cells are very sensitive to heat exposure. This effect is
increased after prolonged hypoxia which induces metabolic changes.
Alterations of glucose metabolism support the action of hyperthermia on hypoxic cells.

Heat exposure interferes with intracellular recovery processes.
At higher temperatures it has a cytotoxic action, at moderate
temperatures the radiosensitization on cells with a high recovery
capacity like melanoma cells is large.

The radiosensitizing effect is mainly caused by interference with radiation induced damage to the chromatin or the cell nucleus and its repair after irradiation.

ACKNOWLEDGEMENTS

The investigations are supported by a grant from the "Bundesminister für Jugend, Familie und Gesundheit", Federal Republic of Germany.

REFERENCES

1. Streffer, C., van Beuningen, D., Dietzel, F., Röttinger, E., Robinson, J.E., Scherer, E., Seeber, S. and Trott, K.-R. (1978). Cancer Therapy by Hyperthermia and Radiation, Urban & Schwarzenberg, Baltimore-Munich.

2. Born, R. and Trott, K.-R. (1978) In: Cancer Therapy by Hyperthermia and Radiation, Urban & Schwarzenberg, Baltimore-Munich, p. 177.

3. Gerweck, L.E., Nygaard, T.G. and Burlett, M. (1979) Cancer Research 39, 966-972.

4. v. Ardenne, M. (1967) Grundlagen der Krebs-Mehrschritt-Therapie. VEB Volk und Gesundheit, Berlin.

5. Streffer, C., Schubert, B., Löhmer, H. and Tamulevicius, P. (1979) In: Thermal Characteristics of Tumors, New York Academy of Sciences (in press).

6. Clark, E.P. and Lett, J.T. (1976) Radiat. Res. 67, 519 (abstracts).

7. Westra, A. and Dewey, W.C. (1971) Int. J. Radiat. Biol. 19, 467-477.

8. Gerweck, L.E., Gilette, E.L. and Dewey, W.C. (1975) Radiat. Res. 64, 611-623.

9. van Beuningen, D., Streffer, C., Zamboglou, N., Schubert, B. and Lindscheid, K.-R. (1979) In: Kombinierte Strahlen- und Chemotherapie, Urban & Schwarzenberg, Baltimore-Munich (in press).

10. Schmidt, W. (1975) Mutation Res. 31, 9-15.

11. Dewey, W.C. and Sapareto, S.A. (1978) In: Cancer Therapy by Hyperthermia and Radiation, Urban & Schwarzenberg, Baltimore-Munich, pp. 149-150.

12. Gerner, E.W. and Schneider, M.J. (1975) Nature (Lond.) 256, 500-502.

13. Henle, K.J. and Leeper, D.B. (1976) Radiat. Res. 66, 505-518.

14. Joshi, D.S. and Jung, H. (1979) Europ. J. Cancer 15, 345-350.

© 1979, Elsevier/North-Holland Biomedical Press
Treatment of Radioresistant Cancers
M. Abe, K. Sakamoto and T.L. Phillips eds.

HYPERTHERMIA IN CANCER THERAPY

R.J.R. Johnson, J.R. Subjeck, H. Kowal, D. Yakar, D. Moreau
Department of Radiation Medicine, Roswell Park Memorial Institute,
666 Elm Street, Buffalo, New York   14263   USA

The oncologists goal is to increase patient survival without an increase in
morbidity. Probably only small increases of 10 to 20 percent can be obtained
by improving local tumor control. Improved treatment cf regional lymph nodes
such as paraaortic nodes in gynecological cancer may not significantly increase
survival since they may be associated with distant metastases. Improved local
tumor control however, will result in an improved quality of survival, and local
hyperthermia in conjunction with small doses of radiation or chemotherapy may
be beneficial in retreating previous radiation failures.

Methods to control metastatic disease are necessary in order to dramatically
improve survival. Currently, chemotherapy alone has not controlled microscopic
metastatic disease except for a few specific tumor types. Whole body hyperthermia in conjuction with other modalities has a yet unknown potential to
control microscopic metastases.

For cancer therapy, hyperthermia may be applied to the whole body, extremity,
thorax, abdomen or a local tumor area. Current biology would suggest that
hyperthermia either applied 48 hours before radiation or 24 hours after
radiation will cause additive damage. Hyperthermia given immediately before,
during or after radiation or chemotherapy may be synergistic in action. The
area required to be treated by hyperthermia will determine whether the combined
modality must improve the therapeutic ratio or only the therapeutic efficacy.
If the clinical requirements dictate use of treatment to regional or whole body
areas it is necessary that hyperthermia be used to cause a greater degree of
cell kill to the tumor than to the normal tissue. If however, hyperthermia is
required for local areas only an increase in the therapeutic ratio may not be
required since the therapeutic efficacy may be improved by differentially
heating the tumor. Differential heating may possibly occur with regional or
whole body heating if energy is preferentially absorbed by the tumor cells,
lost at a decreased rate by the tumor region or produced at a greater rate by
tumor metabolism.

Potential methods available for increasing the therapeutic efficacy include
engineering advances to localize tumor heat production or cooling normal tissue

together with body mechanisms available to differently cool normal tissue.

For hyperthermia to improve the therapeutic ratio when used with either chemotherapy or radiation it is necessary for the in vivo tumor cells to be more sensitive to the application of the heat than the normal tissue and for the synergistic effect of the hyperthermia to be greater on the tumor cells.

The development of hyperthermia as a cancer modality requires the investigation of (1) the biological factors associated with hyperthermia; (2) information on any secondary physiological changes which occur in normal tissue and tumor; and (3) design and testing of both heating modalities and temperature control systems.

BIOLOGICAL RESPONSE TO THERMAL STRESS

As with ionizing radiation, thermal damage of sufficient magnitude will result in cell death. The mechanism for thermal inactivation is unknown, although denaturation of critical chromosomal proteins, polymerases, etc. and/or (phase) changes in cell membranes at a supramolecular level may be involved. Such an effect may result in genetic damage or damage to membrane transport systems with posssible osmotic effects.

In vitro studies of cell lines have been used to examine the effect of hyperthermia on "normal" and corresponding virally transformed cultures, the latter exhibiting a "malignant" potential in host animals. These studies have demonstrated no consistent differences in the sensitivity of these "normal" and "malignant" system to hyperthermia. The association of membrane fluidity and sensitivity to thermal insult [1] would suggest such an association, should the cells plasma membrane represent a primary target for damage.

An Arrhenius plot for heat inactivation of cultured mammalian cells suggests that two independent mechanisms for cell killing may exist, one above and the other approximately below $43^{\circ}C$ [2]. This phenomena corresponds to several observations concerning alterations in the behavior of cells to thermal stress above and below this temperature. Interpretation of cell response should be viewed in light of two potentially different mechanisms for damage.

One observation which illustrates a change in response around $43^{\circ}C$ is thermal tolerance [2]. At temperatures in excess of $43^{\circ}C$ a negative exponential relationship between cell survival and time of thermal exposure exists. This is similar to the effect of ionizing radiation on cell survival. However, at temperatures below $43^{\circ}C$ which are still potentially lethal to many cells, a level of survival is attained in an exponential manner with exposure time, beyond which subsequent thermal exposure has little or no effect. These surviving cells have achieved a tolerance to additional thermal challenge. It is possible that the mechanism of inactivation which occurs at temperatures below $43^{\circ}C$ as demonstrated by an Arrhenius plot is related to the cells ability to develop tolerance in this same temperature range. The ability of the cell to potentially cope with this kind of inactivation may suggest a "competitive repair" process for this damage. At higher temperature (above 43°) damage becomes either overwhelming or of a completely differently, nonrepairable nature.

Thermal tolerance is not a permanent phenomena if cells are returned to $37^{\circ}C$, but disappears after a period of 36 to 72 hours at this temperature. This fact becomes of immediate clinical importance in timing subsequent doses of hyper- thermia in cancer therapy. Present data suggest that hyperthermia treatment should be spaced by not less than 72 hours to allow for recovery from thermal tolerance. This parameter is not yet clearly defined and the recovery time for normal and malignant cells may not be the same. The therapeutic ratio could theoretically be improved by selecting the treatment interval if normal cell's thermal tolerance was longer than tolerance of the tumor cells.

Studies involving hyperthermia of synchronized cultures of cells indicate a cell cycle effect [3]. Cells in the S phase of the mitotic cycle suffer a greatly enhanced susceptability to thermal damage compared to other periods of the cell cycle. This feature is again of clinical interest since S phase is specifically resistant to damage by x rays. This suggests a valuable complementary associa- tion between hyperthermia and x rays in the treatment of cancer.

In addition to this attractive complementary interaction, hyperthermia exhibits an enhanced ability to damage hypoxic tumor regions which are specific- ally resistant to x rays due to the absence of oxygen (a radiation sensitizer) in these regions. When tumor growth removes regions of tumor to distances exceeding 150 to 200 μ from the hypoxia and eventual necrosis occur [4]. Under hypoxic conditions cell metabolism relies greatly on anerobic pathways with subsequent lactic acid buildup and a reduction in pH. It has been demon- strated that a decrease in a few tenths of pH unit greatly increases the likei- hood that cell death will occur in the presence of a given hyperthermia dose [5]. For these reasons hypoxic cells which are resistant to x rays are likely to be more sensitive to hyperthermia.

Tumor hyperthermia applied either at 41.5 to $42^{\circ}C$ or 42.5° to $44.5^{\circ}C$ immedi- ately before radiation may either increase or decrease the radiation response by either decreasing or increasing the hypoxic tumor cell fraction. An increase in the radiation response might also be observed in normal tissues which exist in marginal radiobiological hypoxic conditions, providing the increased blood flow is not offset by corresponding increase in metabolism. Dickson and

Suzangar [6] have reported that 54 of 161 slides obtained from a variety of solid human cancers have a significant inhibition of respiration following 4 hours at $42^\circ C$, whereas, only 3 of 74 normal tissue slides showed inhibition or respiration at this temperature. Temperatures above $42^\circ C$ will progressively decrease the metabolic rate for both tumor and normal tissue. Durand using an in vitro study has reported temperatures of $41^\circ C$ initally cause an increase in oxygen utilization, which subsequently is followed by a decrease in oxygen consumption [7]. The overall effect cf hyperthermia either at 42 or $44^\circ C$ on the tumor hypoxic cell fraction will depend on both the altered rate of oxygen consumption and on changes in oxygen supply.

Tissue is a poor conductor of heat and heat transfer in the body is predominately dependent on ability of the organisms circulatory system to remove heat from a given region. Hypoxic and necrotic regions of a tumor with poor circulation would be expected to contain heat more effectively and reach higher temperatures than well vascularized normal tissue in a given hyperthermia treatment.

The above radiobiological factors project an attractive relationship between radiation therapy and hyperthermia. Application of localized hyperthermia during chemotherapy may also yield beneficial results since transport of the chemotherapeutic agent to the tumor relative to normal tissue may be increased.

Another interesting question in either electromagnetically or ultrasonically induced hyperthermia is whether the effect is identical to simple conduction heating or whether additional perturbations are present. Cavitation effects in ultrasound are an example of such an influence. Some laboratories have claimed an enhancement in vivo tumor response in the presence of electromagnetic heating relative to water bath under comparable, thermal conditions [8]. Other studies have indicated that in vitro microwaves hyperthermia may be dissimilar to water bath heating [9,10]. Preliminary data suggests that heating with 915 MHz microwaves may significantly reduce cell survival relative to waterbath heating at time intervals in excess of approximately 40 min. The difficulty in either in vivo or in vitro studies of this nature center on the difficulty in achieving precise thermometry in electromagnetic fields. However, if such observations are substantiated it may be possible to achieve a temperature bonus, that is cell survival effects characteristics of 42.5 at a fraction of a degree lower temperature.

METHODS AND RESULTS

LeVeen et al [11] and Hahn [12] have used RF Heating at a frequency of 13.56v MHz applied to the patient by surface electrodes. LeVeen states that temperatures exceeding $46^\circ C$ were always achieved in tumors, due to decreased blood flow present in the tumors examined. Many of the tumors treated were exposed at the time of surgery. Very limited data on thermometry were reported. Hahn reports[12] that radiofrequency current hyperthermia may provide good heat distributions for some tumors, since the surface electrodes can be shaped to obtain the desired distribution. The method appears to have limitations, due to fall-off heat at depth and from excessive surface heating the latter of which might be alleviated by controlling the temperature of the surface plates by cooling. Sternhagen et al[13] reported on the use of localized current field at 500 KHz using either non-invasive exterior electrodes or implanted needle electrodes in five patients with recurrent tumors. Hyperthermia was applied without radiation therapy and tumor regression was reported using temperatures of 44°C. Brenner and Yerushalami[14] reported on 6 patients treated by simultaneous heating and radiation applied, at the end of the 45 to 60 minute heating period. Heat was applied initally using hot water; later microwaves were used. Skin temperatures at 42 to 48°C were stated to occur during microwave heating. The authors reported good tumor regression with an increase in the normal skin response.

Johnson et al[15] reported a pilot study of radiation and hyperthermia performed to develop a method to obtain the therapeutic ratio for combined radiation with whole body hyperthermia at 41.5 to 42°C. This study used multiple cutaneous metastatic human tumors, which were treated with a range of radiation doses with higher dose fractions given without heat, while for the low dose fractions both the tumor and skin were heated to 41.5 to 42°C. Heat was applied using 915 MHz micorwaves. Either liquid dielectric or air surface cooling was developed for use with 915 MHz in order to obtain an improved heat distribution at depth. Results from the pilot study suggest a thermal temperature enhancement ratio for tumors 1.2 to 1.3. The skin scoring data for normal tissue thermal enhancement ratio was inadequate in the pilot study to obtain a therapeutic ratio; however, it was apparent that the normal skin response was increased by the addition of post radiation hyperthermia. A cooperative group protocol has been developed by RTOG to establish a therapeutic ratio for post radiation heating of tumor and skin to 41.4 to 42°C using a heat period of 2 hours and 3 radiation fractions with 72 hours between each fraction to avoid thermal tolerance.

In vivo studies on a pig system have been performed by Kowal et al[16] to further evaluate temperature distributions at a depth in tissue. A comparative study of 915 and 434 MHz was made with and without surface cooling. Surface cooling was performed by passing cool air through pores on the face of an adaptor fitted to the microwave applicator, onto the skin of the treatment area.

76

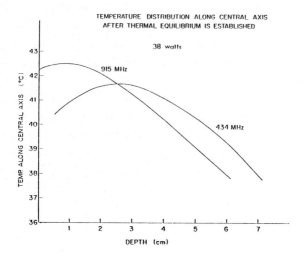

Figure 1   Thermal depth dose in the pig without skin cooling.

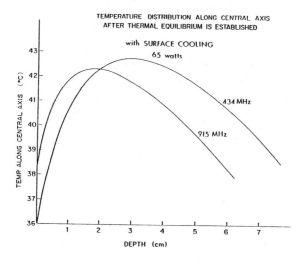

Figure 2   Thermal depth dose in the pig with skin cooling. Skin cooling
allows the application of increased power while not exceeding
acceptable temperatures in the tissue.

Skin temperatures during exposure of 35.8 to 38.4°C were maintained. The results obtained from these studies showed that tissue could effectively be
heated up to a depth of approximately 5 cm (fig 1) at 434 MHz without surface
cooling, and without exceeding a temperature of 42.5°C at any point. With
surface cooling (fig 2) tissue up to a depth of 6.8 cm can be heated and temperature distributions between 2 cm and 6 cm could maintain within ± 1°C of 41.
5°C. With surface cooling 434 MHz produces equivalent heating to 915 MHz, but
at 1.5 cm to 2.0 cm increased depth. In another set of experiments the temperature of the cooling air further reduced by intially passing it over dry ice.
Skin temperature of 20° to 22°C were obtained in this case during exposure.
In this case a constant treatment temperature was found to occur at 915 MHz between 1.0 to 5.5 cm at desired treatment temperatures. This type of cooling
with 434 MHz produced an effect analagous to fig 2.

Hahn [12] has developed an ultrasound technique using surface cooling of the
skin. He has obtained, in human tumors, temperatures of 43.5°C at 3 cm depth
with skin temperatures of 41°C. Storm at al [17] at UCLA developed a "magnetrode"
to inductively heat tumor with frequency of 13.56 MHz. Dr. Storm states that
temperatures of 50°C can be obtained in a tumor located any where in the body.

THE USE OF 434 MHZ MICROWAVES

Holt reported [18] excellent results using 434 MHz microwaves with radiation.
The microwaves were produced by multiple Siemens Units with airwave guides ar-
ranged to form a tunnel around the patient. Microwaves were administered post
radiation for approximately 30 minutes. Tumor and skin temperatures were not
monitored. The radiation was supplied in moderate size fractions.

Hornback [19] acquired similar units and also reported promising results. More
recently Caldwell purchased the 434 MHz Units. He attempted to make thermal
measurements in pigs and in man. The airwave guides caused such interference
with metal temperature measurement probes that temperature measurements could
only be made by inserting the probes through cathetors immediately after the
units were switched off. Deep temperatures of 39-41.5°C were recorded.

At Roswell Patk an _in vitro_, _in vivo_ and clinical study of 434 MHz hyperthermia is being performed to clarify the optimistic clinical reports of 434 MHz
hyperthermia by Dr. Holt and Dr. Hornback.

To simulate clinical conditions the effect of microwave hyperthermia on V 79
cell survival is being investigated with and without radiation, using microwaves
at a measured temperature of 41°C compared with waterbath controls heated to same
temperature. Preliminary results at 915 MHz show that cell survival can be
significantly decreased by high microwave powers and measured temperatures of

41°C compared with 41°C waterbath conditions at exposure times of 60 minutes. The magnitude of this "nonthermal" effect is presently being investigated at 434 MHz. Thermal distributions for 434 MHz microwaves have been obtained in pigs both with and without skin cooling. Temperature distributions demonstrated that 434 MHz is superior to 915 MHz as detailed above. The clinical thermal distributions in patients have been shown to be more variable than in swine. Homogenous heating may be maintained in some patients 5 cm in depth. The clinical study investigates post radiation 434 MHz hyperthermia with surface cooling on patients with multiple metastases. Radiation doses of 100 rads to 400 rads are used with post radiation hyperthermia of 41°C in order to simulate Dr. Holt's studies.

The response of the lesions heated to 41°C post radiation has generally been superior to the controls but more patients are required to quantitate the improvement.

WHOLE BODY HYPERTHERMIA

Von Ardenne et al[20] have reported the use of waterbaths for heating patients and have maintained patients at 41.5°C with this method. Although Von Ardenne reported the joint use of radiotherapy and hyperthermia, their method cannot be adapted for simultaneous use of radiotherapy and hyperthermia.

Pettigrew et al[21] initiated the use of heated anesthetic gases together with a surface wax coating to minimize heat loss. This method was modified by Larkin et al[22] who replaced the wax coating with a plastic sheet heated with a temperature controlled blanket. The anesthetic method has the disadvantages of requiring full anesthesia and a heating time of 60 to 90 minutes. Other systems reported include the Siemens Cabinets which used a radiofrequency mattress as an inital boosting procedure. A water heated sleeping bag has been developed by Atkinson et al[23] which has been tested at the National Cancer Institute by Bull and her associates. An extra corporal heating system has been devloped by Parks. The method is claimed to provide more accurate temperature control and faster heating times.

Although Von Ardenne et al[20], Pettigrew et al[21], and Larkin et al[22] have frequently employed radiotherapy at some time period, there has not been a planned controlled study of whole body hyperthermia and radiotherapy. The clinical results from these investigators suggests that the thermal effect of 41.5 to 42°C hyperthermia causes tumor shrinkage with relief of pain and a general improvement in the patients condition.

COMPLICATIONS OF WHOLE BODY HYPERTHERMIA

Physiological monitoring of cardiac output by Atkinson et al[23] shows that the cardiac output must increase several times in order to compensate for the general vasodilatation which occurs when patients are heated under slight anesthesia using katamine. Pettigrew et al [21] reported that heart rate and blood pressure remained within tolerable limits as long as the patient was well anesthetized. Pettigrew reported that the use of dry gases has prevented alveolitis. Larkin et al [22] have reported superficial burns at pressure points from the use of the heated blanket. Unreported experiments in Europe with Siemens Cabinets suggest that patients may be heated without the use of anesthesia. Disseminated intravascular coagulation (D.I.C.) is not infrequently seen in advanced cancer patients undergoing chemotherapy. Ludgate et al [24] reported that there was evidence of D.I.C. in patients with responsive tumors treated with whole body hyperthermia. Three such patients died with platelet counts below 10×10^9/L fibrin-fibrogen degradation product levels of 160, 640 and 160 m/L respectively.

METASTATSES IN THE HYPERTHERMIA PATIENT

Dickson and Muckle have reported [25] that the metastases rate of the VX-2 carcinoma in the rabbit may be increased by hyperthermia, possibly due to an immune process. Yershalami [26] has developed a model system using C3H mice with a Lewis carcinoma which metastasized to the lung. He reports that the appearance of metastases was advanced in the whole body heated animals, whereas there was a delay in the metastases appearance in animals which received effective local hyperthermia treatment.

No clinical data is available on the effect of either regional or whole body hyperthermia on the metastases rate in man, since the majority of patients in which hyperthermia has been used have already been metastatic. Caution should be used before data from animals systems which show immune responses are extrapolated to man. Regional hyperthermia will cause vasodilatation, which may theoretically increase the number of circulation tumor cells however, there is no evidence that the human rate of metastases is directly related to the number of circulating tumor cells.

FUTURE PROSPECTS FOR CLINICAL HYPERTHERMIA

Current results from the use of local clinical hyperthermia confirm that when the hyperthermia is applied immediately before or after radiation that a thermal enhancement ratio (TER) of 1.2 - 1.6 will be obtained. The TER will depend on the temperature and the length of exposure. Insufficient data is available to determine whether in fact the thermal enhancement ratio for the tumor is greater than that for skin when the temperatures are identical. The future use of different time intervals between treatments may improve the therapeutic ratio.

Investigators using both ultrasound, microwave and interstitial RF heating have demonstrated that tumors of certain pathology and in certain sites may be differently heated above that of the surrounding tissue because of a decreased tumor blood flow. The therapeutic efficacy for heat and radiation will be increased for these tumors. Some tumors investigated show an equal or higher rate of blood flow than the normal tissue. In these patients the tumor may be at a lower temperature than the normal tissue and thus would not be differently effected by the radiation.

With the present equipment available, hyperthermia is indicated for those patients where differential heating can be obtained, such as metastatic lymph nodes which lie within five centimeters of the skin's surface. Further improvements in the therapeutic efficacy may be obtained when radiation sensitizers are added to local hyperthermia.

Heating methods and thermometry require further development if deep tumors in the thorax and abdomen are to be heated. LeVeen and Storm both have the ability to heat deep tumors. Hahn and Lele have developed focused ultrasound which may be excellent in heating at depth providing air cavities are absent.

434 MHz microwaves, may not be sufficient to raise the temperature of a deep tumor above $40^{\circ}C$. Further in vitro and in vivo work is also required to determine if electromagnetic and/or ultrasonic heating produce effects which are different from simple water bath heating.

Techniques have been developed to apply whole body hyperthermia safely. Results from whole body hyperthermia alone suggest palliation only. Initial results of whole body hyperthermia and chemotherapeutic agents warn of possible toxicities which may occur. The use of local hyperthermia with chemotherapy for multiple superficial lesions will determine whether in fact the action of the two methods are additive or synergistic. If specific tumor types respond to combined hyperthermia and chemotherapy then it would appear appropriate to proceed with whole body hyperthermia and the same chemotherapy providing toxicity tests have been performed in large animals and phase I human studies.

The great current interest in hyperthermia should lead to rapid development both in equipment and clinical experience which should move the use of hyperthermia from the experimental laboratory into the clinical setting.

ACKNOWLEDGEMENT

This investigation was supported by NCI's Grant Numbers Ca 17609 and Ca 14058-06 awarded by the National Cancer Institute, DHEW.

REFERENCES

1. Dennis, W.H. and Yatkin, M.B. (1978) Abstract, 26th Annual Meeting of the Radiation Research Society, Toronto, Canada, p.53.

2. Dewey, W.C., Hopwood, L.E., Sapareto, S.A., and Gerweck, L.E., (1977) Radiology, 123, 463-474.

3. Westra, A. and Dewey, W.C. (1971) Int. J. Radiat. Biol., 19, 467-474.

4. Thomlinson, R.H. and Gray, L.H., (1955) Br. J. Cancer, 9, 539.

5. Gerweck, L.E. (1977) Radiat. Res., 70,224.

6. Dickson, J.A. and Suzanger, M.A. (1976) Clin. Oncology, 2,141-155.

7. Durand, R.E. (1977) Abstract, 25th Annual Meeting of the Radiation Research Society, San Juan Puerto, Rico, p.29.

8. Marmor, J.B. Hahn, N. and Hahn, G.M. (1977) Cancer Res., 37, 879-883.

9. Subjeck, J. R., Hetzel, F., Sandhu, T.S., Johnson, R.J.R. and Kowal, H. (1978) Abstract, 26th Annual Meeting of the Radiation Research Society, Toronto, Canada, p.128.

10. Li, G., Van Kersen, I., White, K., Hahn, G., Tanabe, E., Vaguine, V. and Williams, N. (1978) Symposium on Electromagnetic Fields in Biological Systems, Ottawa, Canada, p. 14.

11. LeVeen, H.H., Wapnick, S., Piccone, V., Falk, G. and Ahmed, N. (1976) JAMA 235, 20, 2197-2224.

12. Hahn, G., Personal Communication.

13. Sternhagen, C.J. and Doss, J.D. (1976) Presented at the American Society of Therapeutic Radiology Annual Meeting, Atlanta, Georgia.

14. Brenner, H.J. and Yerushalami, A. (1975) Brit. J. Cancer, 33 91-95.

15. Johnson, R.J.R., Sandhu, T.S., Hetzel, F.W. Song, S., Bicher, H., Subjeck J.R., and Kowal, H. Radiat Oncol: Biol. Phys., in press.

16. Kowal, H., Subjeck, J., Kantor, P., Johnson, R.J.R. and McGarry, M. (1979) Conference on Thermal Characteristics of Tumors, New York Acad. Sci., in press.

17. Storm, F.K. (1979) Conference on Thermal Characteristics of Tumors, New York Acad. Sci., in press.

18. Hoh, J.A.C., (1977) Sensitizers and Hyperthermia, Madison, Wisconsin.

19. Hornback, N.B., Shupe, R.E., Shidnia, H., Joe, B.T., Sayoc, E. and Marshall, C. (1977) Cancer, 40, 2854-2863.

20. Von Ardenne, M. Elsner, J., Kruger, W., Reitnauer, P.G. and Rieger, E., (1966) Klin. Wschr., 44, 503-511.

21. Pettigrew, R.T., Galt, J.M., Ludgate, C.M. and Smith, A.N. (1974) Brit. Med. J., 21, 679-682.

22. Larkin, J.M., Edwards, W.S. and Smith, D.E. (1976) Surgical Forum XXVII, 121-122.

23. Atkinson et al; Personal Communication.

24. Ludgate, C.M., Webber, R.G., Pettigrew, R.T. and Smith, A.N. (1976) Clin. Oncology, 2, 219-225.

25. Dickson, J.A., and Muckle, D.S. (1972) Cancer Res., 32, p. 1916.

26. Yerushalami, A. (1976) Europ. J. Cancer, 12, 455-463.

HIGH LET RADIATION

© 1979, Elsevier/North-Holland Biomedical Press
Treatment of Radioresistant Cancers
M. Abe, K. Sakamoto and T.L. Phillips eds.

BIOLOGICAL PROPERTIES OF FAST NEUTRONS AND NEGATIVE PI-MESONS

K. SAKAMOTO, N. NAKAMURA, Y. TAKAI, S. OKADA

Department of Radiation Biophysics, Faculty of Medicine, University of Tokyo,

Hongo 7-3-1, Bunkyo-ku, Tokyo 113, Japan

S. SUZUKI

Department of Radiology, Institute of Medical Science, University of Tokyo,

Shiroganedai 4-6-1, Minato-ku, Tokyo 108, Japan

INTRODUCTION

Since thirty years, heavy particles such as fast neutrons, negative pi-mesons
and heavy ions were suggested to be introduced to radiotherapy of cancers.
However, there were no accelerators which can be used in particle radiotherapy
because of their inadequate beam intensities and beam energies. Recently fast
neutrons are already used clinically in more than ten facilities in the world.
The pion-therapy has already started at Los Alamos Meson Physics Facility as
test study and radiotherapy with heavy ions is going to start at Lawrence
Berkeley Laboratory.

In these five years, we have been studying the biological effects of fast
neutrons produced from the cyclotron of Institute of Medical Science, University of Tokyo and of negative pi-mesons produced at the TRIUMF cyclotron in
Vancouver. In present paper, relative biological effectiveness (RBE) of fast
neutrons for cultured L5178Y cells and Chinese hamster cells V-79, Elkind recovery of Chinese hamster cells exposed to X-ray or fast neutrons, mutation
frequency induced in L5178Y cells irradiated with X-rays or fast neutrons, RBE
and Oxygen Enhancement Ratio (OER) of fast neutrons and negative pi-mesons for
murine epithelioma and repair of potentially lethal damage of epithelioma cells
exposed to X-rays, fast neutrons and negative pi-mesons are demonstrated.

MATERIALS AND METHODS

Cells and their cultivation. L5178Y cells : Mouse L5178Y cells were cloned
and stored in liquid nitrogen. One ampulla from a cloned population was thawed
and used for each set of the experiments to maintain a relatively low background mutation frequency. Cells were cultured in Fischer's medium containing
100 units/ml of penicillin and 100 μg/ml of streptomycin sulfate.

Chinese hamster cells V-79 : A number of subclones of Chinese hamster cells
designated originally V-79-1 by Elkind has been used. Chinese hamster cells

were cultivated in a modified Eagle's medium to which 15 per cent fetal calf serum was added (EM-15).

Colony formation and mutation assay. Mouse L5178Y cells exposed to radiation were divided into three groups. One group was subjected for colony formation in soft agar containing FM15 (Fischer's medium + 15% of horse serum) in order to estimate its surviving fraction. The second group was incubated in FM10 (Fischer's medium + 10% of horse serum) for six days of the expression time and plated for colony formation in FM15 containing 6-thioguanine (5µg/ml) and soft agar. The third group was incubated in FM10 for three days of the expression time and plated in FM15 containing methotrexate (0.10µg/ml) and soft agar. The number of colonies was scored after 2 weeks. The methods for colony formation for estimation of a surviving fraction, and for mutation frequencies were reported elsewhere[1].

Colony-forming ability was also used in Chinese hamster cells as a measure of the cell's survival in vitro. Cells plated in appropriate numbers in 6 cm petri dishes were grown overnight in a CO_2 incubator at 37°C before experiment was started. During this overnight growth period, initially single cells formed micro-colonies, on average about three cells; consequently the experiments started with populations of micro-colonies rather than single cells. Following irradiation, cells were incubated long enough for a maximum yield of colonies after changing to fresh media. They were then stained with methylene blue and counted.

Mice and tumor. Male and female mice of strain WHT/Ht mice were used as tumor hosts and the tumor used in the experiments was a squamous carcinoma which arose spontaneously in a WHT/Ht albino mice and has since been maintained by serial isologous transplantation as a subcutaneous tumor.

Mice exposed to irradiation were bearing a subcutaneous tumor in each axillary region grown from an inoculum of 50,000 tumor cells injected 10-12 days previously; tumors grew 0.7 cm in diameter at the time of exposure. Single-cell suspensions of tumor cells were prepared from the tumors, transplantation assays of counted suspensions were performed by the technique described by Hewitt et al. using the same tumor[2]. The TD50 (number of cells required for successful transplantation to half a group of injected sites) and its 95 per cent confidence limits were calculated from the results of an assay by the method of Litchfield and Wilcoxon[3].

IRRADIATION

X-irradiation. X-rays were generated by a X-rays therapy machine operated at 200 kVp and 20 mA and were filtrated through 0.5 mm Cu and 1.0 mm Al for _in vitro_ experiments and at 250 kVp and 20 mA using filter of 0.5 mm Cu and 1.0 mm Al for _in vivo_ experiments. Exposure dose rates are 60 rad/min in experiments of cultured cells and 56 rad/min in animal experiments.

Single unanaesthetized tumor-bearing mice were exposed to whole-body irradiation while confined in a perforated Perspex cylinder. For anoxic irradiation, the tumor-bearing mice were killed by nitrogen gas inhalation or neck dislocation and irradiated immediately after death.

Fast neutrons. The fast neutron is produced by bombarding a beryllium target with 15 MeV deuterons extracted from a cyclotron at IMS. Its average energy is 6 MeV. The dose rate was 20 rad/min.

Negative pi-meson beam. The negative pi-meson is produced by bombarding a beryllium target with 500 MeV protons extracted from an isochronous cyclotron at TRIUMF. The dose rate at the pion peak was 2-3 rad/min, and the beam contamination was $\mu^- = 9\%$, and $e^- = 45\%$ by number as determined by time of flight analysis. The pion beam was concentrated over and area of approximately 4 x 4 cm^2, and the tumors were irradiated at the proximal or distal peak of depth-dose curve (Peak I or Peak II) and at the plateau region before or after the peak in depth-dose distribution (Plateau I or Plateau II) of pion beam as shown Fig. 1.

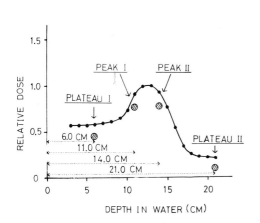

Fig.1 : Depth-dose distribution of pion beam in water phantom. Tumors are situated in the positions (peak I, peak II, plateau I and plateau II) as suggested by circles.

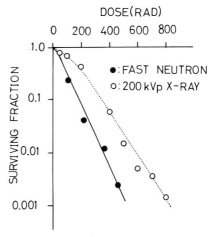

Fig.2 : Single dose survival curves of L5178Y cells exposed to 200 kVp X-rays and fast neutrons.

RESULTS

  Survivals of cultured mammalian cells. Survivals of cultured L5178Y cells
and Chinese hamster cells were determined by colony forming ability of cells.
L5178Y cells usually show small value of D_0 compared with Chinese hamster cells
V-79. The survival curves of L5178Y cells exposed to X-rays and fast neutrons
showed in Fig. 2. D_0s of X-rays and fast neutrons are 110 rad and 70 rad
respectively from the survival curves.

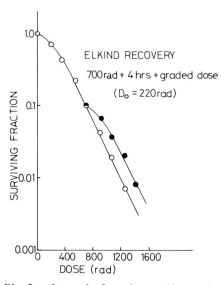

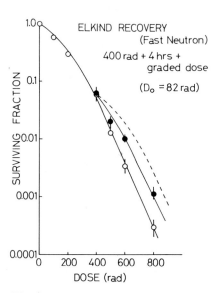

Fig.3 : Open circles show cell survivals
exposed to single doses of X-rays
closed circles show Elking recovery.

Fig.4 : Open circles show cell survivals exposed to fast neutrons,
closed circles show Elkind recovery.

  In Fig. 3 X-ray survival curve of Chinese hamster cells V-79 is shown and the
open circles suggest the surviving fractions of cells irradiated by single doses.
The closed circles demonstrate survivals of cells exposed to graded doses of
X-rays at 4 hours after the first 700 rad irradiation. The cells show full recovery within 4 hours between the first dose and the second dose. The D_0 of
Chinese hamster cells to X-rays is 220 rad, this value is 2 times higher than
that of L5178Y cells. The survival curve of Chinese hamster cells V-79 irradiated with fast neutrons is shown in Fig. 4. The open circles trace the single
dose survival curve of fast neutrons and the closed circles suggest the survivals of cells given graded dose after 4 hours of the first 400 rad. The dotted
line show full recovery curve. From these curves, Chinese hamster cells V-79
irradiated with fast neutrons shows Elkind recovery, but its extent is almost

a half in surviving fraction compared with full recovery. D_O of fast neutrons is 82 rad.

Endpoint	RBE	
	L5178Y cells	V-79 cells
At surviving fraction of 0.1	1.9	2.2
At surviving fraction of 0.01	1.7	2.1

Table 1 : RBEs of fast neutrons calculated from the surviving fractions of L5178Y cells and Chinese hamster cells V-79 exposed to fast neutrons.

RBE values of fast neutrons calculated these results are shown in Table 1, namely 1.6 for L5178Y cells and 2.7 for Chinese hamster cells from the linear slopes of survival curves of cells exposed to X-rays or fast neutrons. The RBEs at the surviving fraction of 0.1 and 0.01 are 1.9, 1.7 for L5178Y cells and 2.2, 2.1 for Chinese hamster cells V-79, respectively.

Mutation frequency of L5178Y cells exposed to fast neutrons. In Fig. 5 mutation frequency of L5178Y cells irradiated with fast neutrons are demonstrated. Mutation frequency is studied by counting drug resistant cell appeared in the media containing 6-thioguanine and methotrexated after irradiation. The dotted line of Fig. 5 is transferred the data obtained with gamma rays of ^{137}Cs from the separate experiments. The left panel of Fig. 5 demonstrates mutation frequency of L5178Y cells investigated using 6-thioguanine as a marker and the right panel shows the results studies using methotrexate as a marker. The mutation frequency induced by fast neutrons increase linearly with dose increment.

In Fig. 6 RBE of fast neutrons to L5178Y cells estimated by various kinds of endpoints, in this figure RBE calculated from appearance of 6-thioguanine resistant cell suggest high RBE value at low dose level and it seemed to decrease with increasing of radiation dose.

Survival curve of murine epithelioma cells irradiated in vivo with X-rays, fast neutrons and pions. Individual mice bearing two tumors were restrained without anaesthesia in a pereforated Perspex cylinder, and surviving fraction of tumor cells were obtained by TD50 assay method. The closed triangles in Fig. 7 trace the survival curve of tumor cells given X-irradiation in vivo under anoxic conditions and the open traiangles or the open circles show the survival of tumor cells irradiated in vivo mice breathing air with X-ray or fast neutrons respectively.

The X-ray survival curve shows two components, and D_Os of the first component

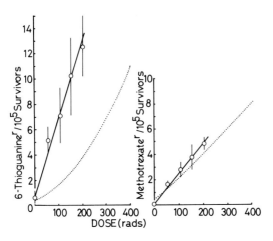

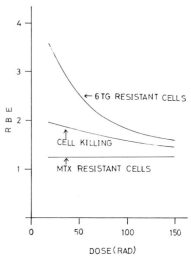

Fig.5 : Mutation frequency of L5178Y cells. The left panel demonstrate mutation frequency studied using 6-thioguanine as a marker. The right panel shows mutation frequency studied using methotrexate as a marker.

Fig.6 : RBEs of fast neutrons to L5178Y cells estimated by various kinds of endpoints.

and the second component are 115 rad and 276 rad. D_0 estimated from the hypoxic cell survival curve is the almost same as that of the second component.

The survival curve obtained by fast neutrons irradiation bends slightly at the surviving fraction of 0.01. D_0 of the first segment is 52 rad and that of the second segment is 99 rad.

The RBEs from the results above-mentioned are summarized in Table 2. The RBEs at the surviving fraction of 0.1, 0.01 and 0.001 are 2.9, 2.8 and 2.8 respectively.

The OERs of X-rays and fast neutrons are 2.4 and 1.9. The OER are estimated assuming that the second component is the anoxic component of a compound curve obtained for the irradiation of mixed population of well-oxygenated and anoxic cells, as described by the theoretical formation of Hewitt and Wilson.

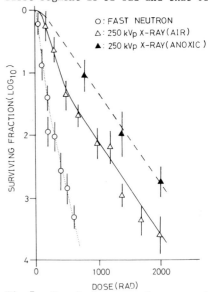

Fig.7 : Survival curve of tumor cells exposed to X-rays or fast neutrons.

Endpoint	RBE
At surviving fraction of 0.1	2.9
At surviving fraction of 0.01	2.8
At Surviving fraction of 0.01	2.8

Table 2 : RBEs of fast neutrons estimated in each survivals fraction of murine epithelioma cells exposed to fast neutrons.

The single-dose survival curve of the squamous carcinoma cells irradiated at the distal peak in depth-dose distribution curve is also demonstrated as a solid line in Fig. 8. The curve which is traced through the open circles bends

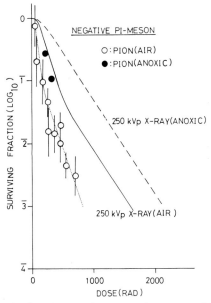
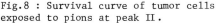
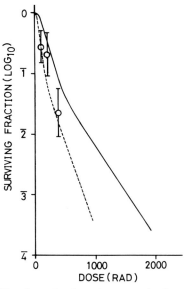

Fig.8 : Survival curve of tumor cells exposed to pions at peak II.

Fig.9 : Circles show survivals of cells exposed to pions at peak I.

slightly at a dose level of around 200 rad. The D_o of the first component is 73 rad and that of the second segment is 130 rad. The closed circles in Fig. 8 suggest the surviving fraction of epithelioma cells irradiated _in vivo_ immediately after killing mice by neck dislocation, and the solid line and the dashed line are superimposed the survival curve of epithelioma cells irradiated with X-rays in air or in anoxic conditions shown in Fig. 7.

The tumor cell survival curve obtained by irradiation at the proximal peak is shown in Fig. 9 and it seems to be the almost same as the curve of the distal peak.

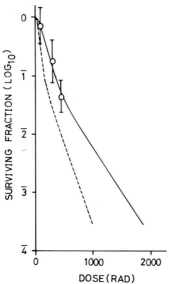

Fig.10 : Circles show survival of cells exposed to pions at plateau I.

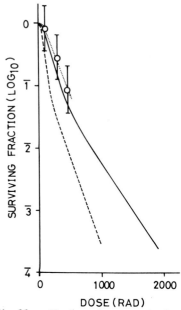

Fig.11 : Circles show survivals of cells exposed to pions at plateau II.

In Fig. 10 the survival curve of tumor cells irradiated at the plateau region before the peak in depth-dose distribution and in Fig. 11 the survival curve of cells at the plateau region after the peak are demonstrated. In Figs. 9, 10 and 11 the dotted line and solid line are transferred from the previous figure shown the effect of pions at the distal peak or 250 kVp X-rays. These results may suggest that the effects of pions at plateau regions to epithelioma cells are the almost same as the effect of X-rays or gamma rays, though experimental points are not so enough.

Endpoint	RBE
At surviving fraction of 0.1	2.2
At surviving fraction of 0.01	2.0

Table 3 : RBEs of pions estimated in each surviving fraction of murine epithelioma cells exposed to pions.

The RBE values of pions obtained from present study are shown Table 3. The RBE's at the surviving fraction of 0.1 and 0.01 are 2.2 and 2.0 respectively.

The oxygen enhancement ratio (OER) is estimated as a ratio of D_0 values of the first component and the second component in each curve, and OER's of X-rays and pion beam are 2.4 and 1.8, if the second component of the survival curves of tumor cells irradiated with pion beam suggests the survival of anoxic cells in tumor like in the case of X-rays.

PLD repair of epithelioma cells. Repair of potentially lethal damage of murine epithelioma cells exposed to X-rays and fast neutrons is studied. To test PLD repair, TD50 assay were performed at various time after irradiation. The results are shown in Fig. 12. The open circles and the closed circles stand for survival of cells at different times after exposure to 1,000 rad and 2,000 rad of X-rays. The closed traiangles suggest cell survivals which is irradiated with fast neutrons, and is assayed at various time after irradiation. The epithelioma cells exposed to X-rays and fast neutrons show the repair of potentially lethal damage, however recovery ratio is almost 60% in fast neutrons compared to X-rays.

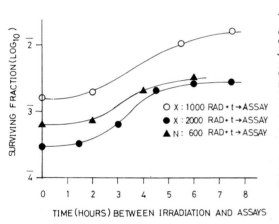

Fig.12 : Curves show repair of potentially lethal damage of murine epithelioma cells irradiated in vivo with X-rays or 1000 rad or 2000 rad and with fast neutrons of 600 rad.

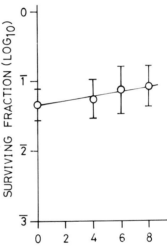

HOURS AFTER IRRADIATION

Fig.13 : PLD repair of murine epithelioma cells exposed to 250 rad of pions at peak II.

The squamous carsinoma were also exposed to 250 rad of pions at the distal peak of the depth-dose distribution curve to study repair of potentially lethal damage. The result is shown in Fig. 13. The epithelioma cells used in the present investigations shows PLD repair slightly after pion irradiation. However, the recovery ratio is smaller than the cells irradiated with X-rays.

DISCUSSION

L5178Y cells are more sensitive to X-rays than Chinese hamster cells V-79, however D_0s of L5178Y cells and Chinese hamster V-79 to fast neutrons are 70 rad and 82 rad, there are no big differences in both cell lines. The RBEs at the surviving fraction of 0.1 and 0.01 are 1.9, 1.7 for L5178Y cells and 2.2, 2.1 for Chinese hamster cells. There are some differences in RBE values between cell lines, it may suggest that fast neutrons is more effective to a radio-resistant cell line.

In Chinese hamster cells exposed to X-rays and fast neutrons Elkind recovery is recognized, however the recovery rate of cells irradiated with fast neutrons is almost a half compared to X-rays. In murine epithelioma, PLD repair is found but the recovery ratio is almost a half in fast neutrons as in Elkind recovery of Chinese hamster cells. These data suggest that in neutron therapy total dose to be required to cure tumors may be able to estimate less than the dose calculated from estimation of RBE only.

In neutron therapy in IMS, 120 rad is used as an individual dose, exposure of 120 rad with fast neutrons to murine epithelioma suggest the surviving fraction of 0.1 and RBE calculated at this surviving fraction is 2.9. On the other hand, mutation frequency of cells exposed to fast neutrons tested using L5178Y cells show the different results by markers, it is difficult to conclude whether or not fast neutrons induce high rate of mutation frequency. However, cells irradiated with fast neutrons may show higher appearance rate of anti-tumor drug resistant cells compared with X-rays.

Concerning RBEs of pions Raju and Richman reviewed RBE values obtained from various pion sources and suggested that the RBE values for pions at the peak line between 1.5-5.0[4]. RBE values depend on the endpoint and biological materials. Mill, Lewis and Hall[5] showed an RBE of 2.1 using HeLa cells, Coggle et al.[6] demonstrated that there are no detectable differences in RBE values among the radiation sources of Cobalt-60 gamma rays, 220 kVp X-rays, 14 MeV X-rays, electrons and pions using various kinds of endpoints like thymic weight loss, oocyte and bone marrow CFU-S survival and induction of macroscopic lens opacities. In our experiment RBE values were calculated to be 2.0 to 2.2 at the peak. These results agree with data presented by other investigators.

The value of OER of pions at the peak were calculated as 1.8 from the survival data of murine epithelioma cells irradiated in vivo. This value is larger than the data of Raju et al.[7]. Raju et al. calculated an OER for pions at the peak to be 1.6 at the 10% surviving level of cultured human kidney cells and 1.9 for reversions to arginine independence in yeast Saccharomyces cervisae.

The value of OER of pions in present paper is obtained as a result of calculation from a ratio of D_0s of the first component and the second component of survival curve, assuming that the second component shows the survival of anoxic cells in tumor. Therefore, if this assumption is wrong the value of OER calculated from the way mentioned above will not be correct. In our experiments the tumor-bearing mice killed by neck dislocation were irradiated with pion beam of 200 rad and 300 rad at the peak, and the surviving fraction of tumor cells showed a little bit higher values compared with the surviving fraction of tumors cells irradiated in air breathing condition, and the line drawn through these two points looks like to show the similar slope as the second component of the tumor cell survival curve of pion beam shown in Fig. 8. However, higher doses must be used for determining the survival curve of anoxic tumor cells, but it was very difficult to do such experiments in present beam conditions at TRIUMF because of low dose rate, as long exposure time would cause autolysis and the other phenomenon in dead mice during exposure.

In fractionated radiotherapy, 200 or 300 rad is usually used as and individual dose, so it seems to be reasonable to compare values at dose level of 200 or 300 rad of 250 kVp X-rays. The dose of pions needed to show the same surviving fraction as obtained by 200 rad irradiation of X-rays is estimated to be 95 rad from the survival curve, and RBE is calculated as 2.2. The effect of pion irradiation of 150 rad to murine epithelioma cells corresponds to the effect of exposure to X-rays of 300 rad, in this case RBE is 2.0.

The X-rays, fast neutrons and pion beam used in the present experiments differ in their dose rate, namely these were 56 rad/min for X-rays, 20 rad/min for fast neutrons, and 2-3 rad/min for pion beam. Therefore, RBE and OER shown here may not express exact values, the experimental results of pions to be obtained by irradiation with higher dose rate than used in present work may show higher RBE value.

ACKNOWLEDGEMENTS

This investigation was supported in part by Japan Society for the Promotion of Sciences.

REFERENCES

1. Knapp, A.G.A.C. and Simons, J.W.I.M. (1975) Mutation Res., 30, 97-110.
2. Hewitt, H.B. et al. (1967) Int. J. Radiat. Biol., 12, 535-549.
3. Litchfield, J.T. and Wilcoxon, F. (1949) J. Pharm. & Exp. Therapy, 96, 99-103
4. Raju, M.R. and Richman, C. (1972) Current Topics in Radiation Research

96

Quarterly, 8, 159–233.

5. Mill, A.J. et al. (1976) Brit. J. Radiol., 49, 166–171.

6. Coggle, J.E. et al. (1976) Brit. J. Radiol., 49, 161–165.

7. Raju, M.R. et al. (1972) Brit. J. Radiol., 45, 178.

© 1979, Elsevier/North-Holland Biomedical Press
Treatment of Radioresistant Cancers
M. Abe, K. Sakamoto and T.L. Phillips eds.

CLINICAL EXPERIENCE WITH CALIFORNIUM-252 BRACHYTHERAPY FOR RADIORESISTANT
TUMORS

KOICHI KANETA, M.D., AKIRA TSUYA, M.D., TAKEO SUGIYAMA, M.D., YOSHIO ONAI,
PH.D*., TEIZO TOMARU, PH.D*., AND TORAJI IRIFUNE, PH.D*.
Department of Radiology, Cancer Institute Hospital and Department of
Physics*, Cancer Institute, Japan

INTRODUCTION

The purpose of this study was to determine the potential advantages of
neutrons produced by nuclear fission of Californium-252 (Cf-252) in treating
radioresistant cancers when compared with radium therapy and also to determine how Cf-252 should be clinically used.

The results of our pilot study with Cf-252 brachytherapy conducted
from March 1974 through December 1978 on 65 cases consisting of 20 primary
cases and 45 secondary cases are summarized and reported here. Small sources
of Cf-252 were made available on loan to the Cancer Institute in 1973 and
also in 1976 from the US Department of Energy (formerly US Energy Research
and Development Administration) under the Cf-252 Market Evaluation Program.

The first loan of 30 ug of Cf-252 small sources consisted of 15 needles
and 6 cells, and the second loan of 87 ug consisted of 10 cells and 16 seed
assemblies.

The details on Cf-252 small sources are presented in Table 1 with their
dimensions.

Before their clinical application, the Physics Department of the Cancer
Institute made studies on the physical properties of Cf-252 and developed
computer assisted dosimetry, various kinds of equipment for radiation
protection, and instruments for safe handling of these sources in therapy[1].
Through their effort clinical application of Cf-252 became possible from
March 1974.

METHOD OF TREATMENT AND SELECTION OF CASES

The method of application was completely comparable to that of Ra small
sources, as they have the same dimensions except for seed assemblies. They
were applied in various forms according to the condition of the disease.
Needles were abandoned since May 1977 due to the high risk of personnel
exposure to neutron radiation. Cells and seed assemblied were used for

manual afterloading, and tubes were used for remotely controlled after-loading unit.

The patient is treated in a special ward with various shielding for personnel protection (Fig. 1).

TABLE 1

CF-252 SMALL SOURCES LOANED TO THE CANCER INSTITUTE HOSPITAL FROM THE US DEPARTMENT OF ENERGY IN OCTOBER 1973 AND IN MARCH 1977

Source type	Active length (mm)	Length (mm)	Capsule wall thickness 90% Pt,10% Ir		External diameter (mm)	Intensity		Number
			inner (mm)	outer (mm)		μg	n/sec.	
Needle, 2.4	30.00 ±0.50	40.00 ±0.50	0.15 ±0.012	0.30 ±0.012	1.65 ±0.025	2.505 ±5.0%	5.800 x10^6	5
Needle, 1.2L	30.00 ±0.50	40.00 ±0.50	0.15 ±0.012	0.30 ±0.012	1.65 ±0.025	1.223 ±5.0%	2.834 x10^6	5
Needle, 1.2S	15.00 ±0.50	26.00 ±0.50	0.15 ±0.012	0.30 ±0.012	1.65 ±0.025	1.256 ±5.0%	2.910 x10^6	5
Short after-loading cell 1.0	15.00 ±0.50	18.00 ±0.50	0.10 ±0.012	0.15 ±0.012	0.99 ±0.025	1.032 ±5.0%	2.391 x10^6	6
Applicator tube	15.00 ±0.50	23.50 ±0.25	0.30 ±0.012	0.50 ±0.012	2.80 ±0.05	15.662 ±5.0%	36.195 x10^6	3
Short after-loading cell	15.00 ±0.50	18.00 ±0.50	10.0 ±0.012	0.16 ±0.012	0.95 ±0.025	0.795 ±5.0%	1.838 x10^6	10
Seed	4.00 ±0.10	6.00 ±0.25		0.16 ±0.012	0.80 ±0.05	0.380 ±5.0%	0.878 x10^6	72

Seed assembly	Active length mm	External length mm	External diameter mm	Number of seeds	Number of seed assemblies
3-seed	26	60	1.05	0.38 μgx3	4
4-seed	36	70	1.05	0.38 μgx4	4
5-seed	46	80	1.05	0.38 μgx5	4
6-seed	56	90	1.05	0.38 μgx6	4

Patients selected for this therapy were classified into 3 groups, for whom conventional radiation therapy was considered to be ineffective.

In the first group were included radioresistant cancers, such as malignant melanoma and differentiated adenocarcinoma of the uterine cervix. In the second group were included esophageal carcinoma and hilar carcinoma of the lung having a high recurrent rate. Included in the third group were recurrent carcinoma following surgery and/or irradiation and residual tumors following irradiation.

As for the method of therapy, 22 cases received direct interstitial theraphy and 15 cases received intracavitary irradiation by manual afterloading main- ly to the esophageal cavity. Twelve cases received interstitial therapy with

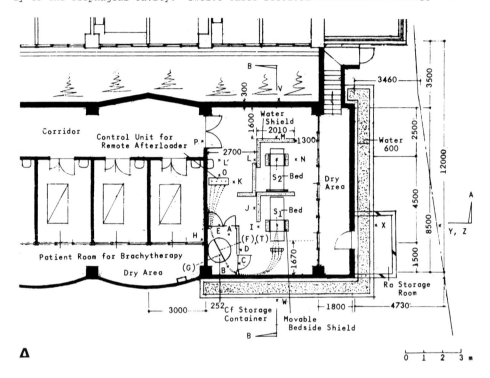

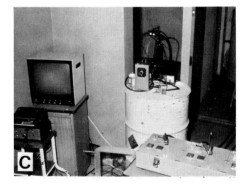
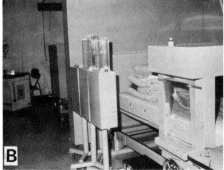

Fig. 1. Diagram of the Cf-252 storage and treatment facility in the treatment room, provided with 2 treatment beds (A). Bed (Sl) in A is used for inter- stitial treatment (B). Control unit for remote afterloader is shown at the lower right corner (C).

seed assemblies by manual afterloading, 6 cases received intracavitary irradiation with remotely controlled afterloading mainly for the bronchus and uterine cavity, and 10 cases received mold therapy. Some of our results has been reported previously[1,2,3].

As mentioned earlier, direct needling was abandoned since 1977, when seed assemblies became available for clinical use.

Our remote afterloader was designed by the Physics Department and constructed in July 1977. This machine is provided with 4 channels, each containing one source to permit independent use. The details of the machine have been reported previously by Onai et al.[4] Some parts of the machine are

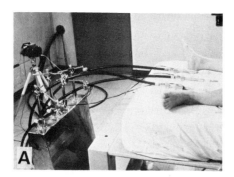
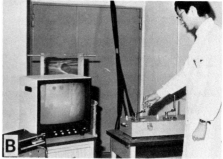
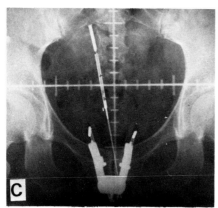
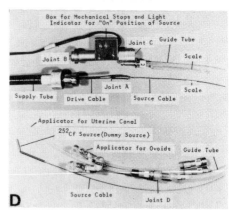

Fig. 2. Cf-252 intracavitary treatment with remote afterloader.
A: Patient being treated.   B: Remote control of the control unit.
C: Orientation film using dummy sources. With the use of the film the
three dimensional dose distribution is computed with a computer.
D: Detailed description of the tip of the 3 channel unit.

shown in Figs. 1 and 2.

We have made some modifications around the tip of the applicator tube of the remote afterloader to facilitate intracavitary application. For bronchial use, a fine tube was attached to the external wall of the applicater tube with the open end at the tip. Local anesthesia is given through this fine tube to the treatment area during treatment.

For esophageal use, a rubber balloon was placed around the tip of the applicator tube. By air inflation of the bulloon the tip is fixed in position, and the clearance and involved esophageal mucosa are expanded, permitting a homogenous irradiation to the tumor. Recently 2 cases were successfully treated with this tube.

Three dimensional dose distribution to the target volume was calculated for both neutrons and γ-rays with a computer using a program developed by Onai et al. for each individual case. The average total target dose of neutrons was aimed at 1200 rad with an assumed RBE value of 6, but it was modified individually according to histology, location, size and condition of the tumor bed, history of surgery, and previous radiotherapy.

RESULTS

Assessment of the therapeutic results was made 2 and 3 months after the completion of therapy, using the early and late effect scores for tumors developed by the National Institute of Radiological Sciences.

They are classified into the following five grades of effectiveness

A: Early effect score of tumor control

    1 --- Complete disappearance of tumor.

    2 --- Regression, less than half of the original size.

    3 --- Regression, larger than half size of the original.

    4 --- No shrinkage.

    5 --- Growing.

B: Late effect score of tumor control

    1 --- Complete disappearance with no sign of scar.

    2 --- Complete disappearance with scar formation.

    3 --- Residual but non-growing tumor.

    4 --- Residual and slowly growing tumor.

    5 --- Rapidly growing recurrent tumor.

The relationship between the local tumor response by early effect score and the number of cases in each group of diseases is shown in Table 2.

The neutron dose was used to represent the absorbed dose, because the γ-ray contribution was considered to be minor from the standpoint of biological effectiveness, when these sourses were applied at a low dose rate, and when it was assumed that the RBE value of fast neutrons released from these sources was sufficiently large, for example 6 or 7.

1. Primary case

Eight primary cases out of 20 were treated solely with Cf-252 (Table 2), and the remaining 12 cases were treated by Linac X-rays or Co-60 γ-rays supplemented with Cf-252 boost therapy.

a) Neutron therapy only :

One case of malignant melanoma of the vagina (Case 13, Fig. 6) was controlled by Cf-252 volume interstitial irradiation of neutron dose of 1440 rad in 6 days. Tumor disappeared completely. She died of other cause 1.5 years later.

TABLE 2

DISTRIBUTION OF TREATED CASES AND EARLY TUMOR EFFECT SCORE

No. of cases assigned		Score		Score 4 or 5 or salvaged by operation	Scoring not possible	Total
		1	2 or 3			
Primary cancer Cf-252 only	Uterine cervix	5(2)*	–	–	1(1)	6(3)
	Vulva	1	–	–	–	1
	Skin	–	1	–	–	1
Cf-252 boost	Tongue	1(1)	–	–	–	1(1)
	Esophagus	1	6	–	–	7
	Skin	1	–	–	–	1
	Lymph node	–	1	–	–	1
	Bronchus	–	1(1)	1(1)	–	2(2)
Recurrent cancer						
Head and neck		13(1)	3(3)	3(1)	4(2)	23(7)
Uterus		4(1)	4	2	–	10(1)
Esophagus		–	2	–	–	2
Skin		2	1	–	–	3
Lung or mediastnum		–	–	1(1)	–	1(1)
Malignant melanoma		1	–	–	–	1
Miscellaneous		2(1)	3(3)	–	–	5(4)
Total		31(6)	22(7)	7(3)	5(3)	65(19)

*
No. of cases treated with seed assembries or remote afterlorder is shown in parentheses.   March 1974 — Dec. 1978

Four cases of well differentiated papillary adenocarcinoma of the cervix uteri (Cases 22, 23, 24 and 53; Figs. 3, 4 and 5) were also treated with intracavitary application of Cf-252. The neutron dose to Point A was 430 to 470 rad in 6 or 20 fractions in 2 months. Local clinical findings and follow-up histological examinations revealed remarkable effectiveness of this therapy especially histologically. Two cases out of 4 are living without disease for 1 or 3 years. Both of them had T1b disease with no regional metastasis and the minimum neutron dose to the target volume was estimated to be 840 rad. Two other cases (Cases 23 and 53) were salvaged by surgical removal due to recurrence 6 months later. These two cases had T3b disease and minimum delivered neutron dose to Point A was estimated to be less than 500 rad. For these cases irradiation was supplemented by Cf-252 manual afterloading applied for corpostat and for tandem.

Until 1977 when the remote afterloader became available for use, Cf-252 needles were bundled to make an intracavitary tandem. Cf-252 cells were used for corpostat. These sources were inserted into the uterine cavity by manual afterloading technique.

Fig. 3 is an example treated with this technique. It is noteworthy that very marked histological changes were soon observed by successive histological examinations (Figs. 4 and 5). One case of adenosquamous carcinoma of the uterine cervix (Case 58, T1bNXMO) was successfully treated with a neutron dose of 1200 rad to the target area (the dose to Point A was 560 rad). In this case, the histological changes were favorable, and there were no cancer cells after delivery of a neutron dose of 600 rad.
She was eventually cured and has been living well for more than one year.

b) Neutron boost therapy :

Twelve primary cases out of 20 were treated by neutron boost therapy, which consisted of 7 cases of esophageal cercinoma, one case each of metastatic lung carcinoma (Case 8) and skin cancer (Case 19), and 2 cases of bronchial cancer (Cases 46 and 63). External irradiation of 5000-7000 rad was given to the esophagus, followed by boost intracanalicular application of Cf-252 for the eradication of the remaining radioresistant nests. Neutron doses of 60 to 260 rad were given to a point 0.5 cm from the center of the tube. For esophageal cancer, results more favorable than those of the external X-irradiated group could not be obtained.

One case of bronchogenic carcinoma and one case of supraclavicular lymph node metastasis of the lung were controlled favorably for 20 months or more than 3 years.

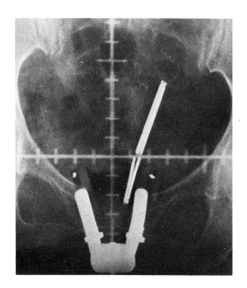 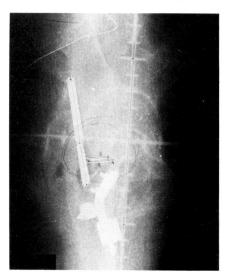

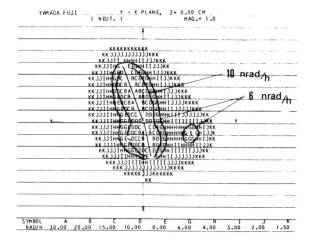

Fig. 3. Case 22. Primary uterine cervix cancer with papillary adenocarcinoma, TlbNXMO. Intracavitary application of 9.7 ug of Cf-252 in tandem and 3.3 ug in corpostat was made for 144 hrs/6F/4 weeks. A neutron dose of 864 rad was given to the target volume. Positioning films taken from two perpendicular directions, (upper panel) and areal dose rate distribution of neutron on the X-Y plane (lower panel).

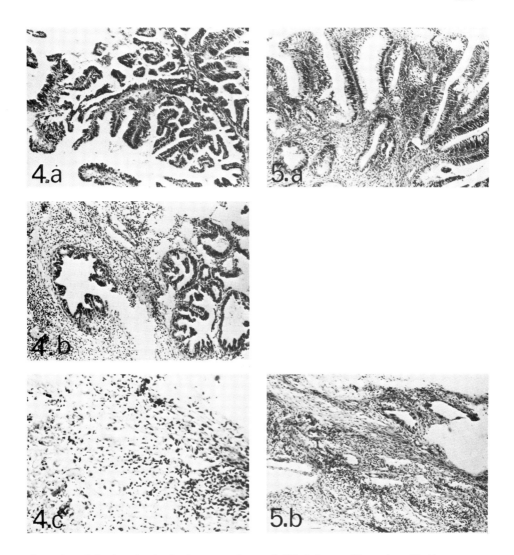

Figs. 4. and 5. Histological changes after Cf-252 intracavitary irradiation.

Fig. 4. Case 22.   Primary uterine cervix cancer with papillary adenocarcinoma, T1bNXM0.   4a: Prior to Cf-252 treatment.   4b: Two days after the 1st session of Cf-252 intracavitary irradiation for 24 hrs.   Almost no change was observed.   4c: Two days after the 3rd session of the treatment.   864 rad/ 6F/4 W was given to the target area.   No cancer cells were seen.   The patient has been living without disease for 3.5 years.

Fig. 5. Case 23.   Primary uterine cervix cancer with papillary adenocarcinoma, T3bNXM0.   432 rad/6F/4 W was given to the target volume.   5a: Prior to therapy. 5b: Marked radiation effect with tiny degenerative cancer foci was seen. The patient received hysterectomy due to recurrence 1 year later and died of generalized matastasis 2.5 years later.

2. Secondary cases

Forty-five secondary cases consisted of 23 cases of head and neck cancer, 10 cases of uterine cervix cancer, 3 cases of skin cancer, one case of suspected mediastinal origin, one case of malignant melanoma, and 5 cases of miscellaneous cancer as shown in Table 2. They were considered to be poor candidates for conventional photon therapy, because they had underwent previous operation and/or irradiation. Thirteen head and neck cases out of 23 have been doing well for more than 1 year. Local control was achieved in 9 out of 13 recurrent cancer cases of the tongue and floor of the mouth for more than 6 months. There were 4 cases whose conditions were found to be suspicious recurrence 5 - 12 months after completion of Cf-252 treatment. All 4 cases were salvaged by operation. In three cases of them (Cases 27, 32 and 43) no cancer cells could be demonstrated in their removed specimens (Fig.9.).

One recurrent tongue cancer case (Case 7) was successfully treated by direct needling and therefore was shown in Fig. 6.

Local control was achieved in 1 case of adenoid cystic carcinoma of the soft palate (Case 36), and in 1 case of malignant melanoma of the ethmoid (Case 34). Three out of 10 cases of uterine cervix cancer showed good early effect (Score 1) but 2 of them recurred after 3 and 6 months, respectively. Two cases of esophageal cancer could not be controlled and one case of skin cancer (Case 29) achieved local control but later developed brain necrosis due to excessive cumulative irradiation. Another skin cancer case (Case 20) underwent surgery because of poor local effect. Local control was achieved in one case of recurrent rectal carcinoma in the perineal region (Case 4).

Recently, 12 cases were treated with Cf-252 seed assemblies by manual afterloading method. One representative case is shown in Fig. 7. She had previous irradiation followed by partial resection and cryosurgery for her tongue cancer. The operation of recurrent tumor was refused. Six seed assemblies were inserted with loop technique by manual afterloading. Initial 84 hours' irradiation was given and the neutron dose rate distribution is shown on the left side of the figure. Second 84 hours' irradiation was given after withdrawal of central 2 seed assemblies in order to obtain homogenous dose distribution throughout the target area.

Total neutron dose of 1680 rad was delivered in 168 hours. She was well for 1 year until suspicious recurrent focus was found. The focus was

removed by surgery.   There was no cancer cells detected in the removed
specimen.   She has been well for more than 1 year after the last operation.

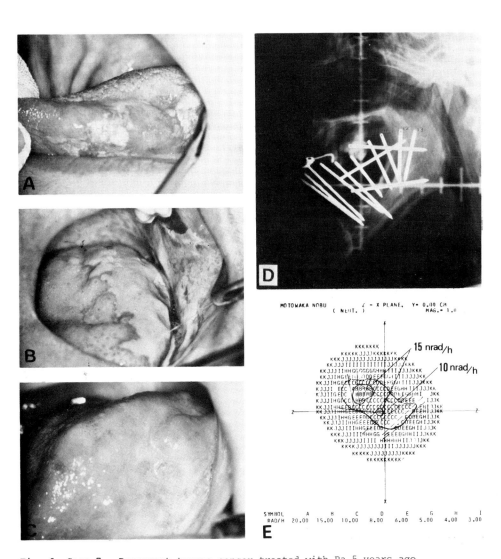

Fig. 6. Case 7. Recurrent tongue cancer treated with Ra 5 years ago.
A: Before Cf-252 treatment. Recurrent foci were seen in previously
treated area of the tongue. Single plane implantation was made for 168
hrs. A neutron dose of 1848 rad was delivered in 168 hrs. to the tumor.
B: Moderate mucocitis continued for 1 year. C: Healed mucocitis.
The patient has been living without disease for 4.5 years. D: Positioning
film taken from lateral side. E: Areal dose rate distribution on the
X-Z plane.

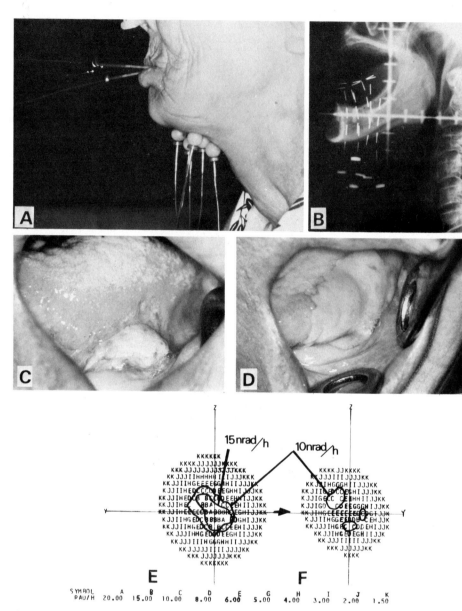

Fig. 7. Case 43. Recurrent carcinoma of the tongue extending to the gingiva.
A: Six seed assemblies were inserted with loop technique by manual afterloading.
B: Positioning film taken from lateral side.
C: Before treatment.
D: After treatment, moderate mucositis was seen.
E: Areal dose rate distribution (six sources).
F: Same as above (after removal of two sources). For details refer to the text.

3. Overall results

It is to be noted that good local control of score 1 was achieved in 30 out of 60 cases as summarized in Table 2. Assessment of the effect was impossible in 5 cases. One case of 5 cases showed generalized matastases during the treatment, one other case died suddenly soon after treatment, and the remaining 3 cases received Cf-252 treatment as postoperative prophylactic irradiation.

Score 1 response was obtained in 52 % or 31/60 of the cases treated, that is, in 58% or 14/24 cases of head and neck tumor, in 17% or 3/18 cases of the thoracic and abdominal region such as esophageal cancer and lung cancer, in 56% or 9/16 of cases of uterine cervix cancer.

This therapy is considered to be most rewarding in the treatment of recurrent cancers of the tongue and the floor of the mouth, most of which will not be salvaged except by radical surgery including removal of the lower jaw.

No significant complication was encountered except in 2 cases (Cases 33 and 65). The former case developed deep ulceration in the mouth floor after irradiation whose dose was considered not to be excessive. The latter case developed ulceration in the perineal region 5 months later. She was treated by the implantation of Cf-252 seed assemblies with a neutron dose of 1500 rad 3 months after the previous Ra implantation for her postoperative recurrent rectal cancer, which was considered to be excessive.

The relationship between delivered neutron dose and local response is shown in Fig. 8.

The delivered neutron dose differed considerably according to disease and conditions.

A minimum neutron dose of more than 600 rad was considered necessary to eradicate the disease [5,6,7,8], although a higher neutron dose is considered necessary and tolerable for the treatment of primary uterine cervix cancer. Poor tolerance of the urinary bladder and rectal mucosa to neutron irradiation was observed in our experience. Results of Cf-252 treament for the recurrent uterine cervix cancer were not rewarding as shown in Figs. 8 and 9, when extensive intracavitary Ra irradiation had been given previously.

4. Survival

The relationship between early tumor effect score and long term results is shown in Fig. 9 according to 3 disease groups. They are 1) primary uterine cervix cancer group (5 cases), 2) recurrent uterine cervix cancer group (10 cases), and 3) recurrent head and neck cancer group (16 cases).

110

Each case treated was classified into one of 6 columns, that is living without disease, living with disease, living after salvage operation for true recurrence, living after salvage operation for false recurrence, died of cancer, and died of other cause.

Judging from Fig. 9, primary uterine cervix cancer group showed the best result, which was followed by recurrent head and neck cancer group.

5. Skin reaction or other side effects

No severe cutaneous or mucosal damage was observed except one case (Case 65) even when the delivered dose exceeded 1500 rad.

A comparison of skin reaction has been made between Ra and Cf-252 in 2 cases to obtain the clinical RBE value.

An example is shown in Fig. 10. The RBE value of 5 to 7 was obtained by comparing the skin response and corresponding absorbed dose profiles.

DISCUSSION

Protection of hospital personnel from neutron exposure is essential for

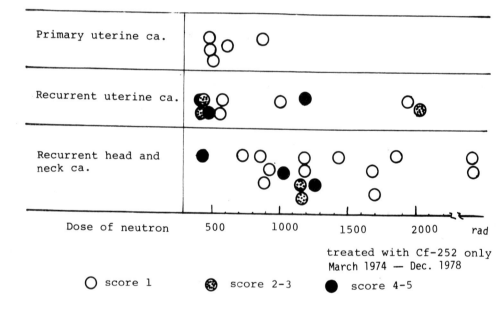

Fig. 8. Distribution of dose delivered and early tumor effect score in cases treated from March 1974 to Dec. 1978

the safe handling of this source. At present, afterloading technique is used in all cases, either manually or by the use of remote afterloading technique. The construction of remote afterloader for interstitial application should facilitate increased use of this therapy in the future. In such a case, if the diameter of the seed assemblies could be made much smaller, maniplation would become far easier.

As seed assemblies are relatively flexible and various length of sources are available, there might be an additional applicability of expanding its indication for deep-seated localized lesions, when combined with surgery.

The superiority of this therapy to various kinds of widely used γ-ray small sources should be confirmed by controlled clinical trials. Uterine cervix cancer, either in advanced stage or of radioresistant histology type, would be the candidate of controlled clinical trials, because of the high incidence of the disease. If this experience proves favorable, this can be made available for a reasonable period of time to a larger number of patients. Cf-252 represents a source which may be advantageously utilized as a replacement for Ra brachytherapy. The search for probable indications constitutes the subject for future clinical trial[9].

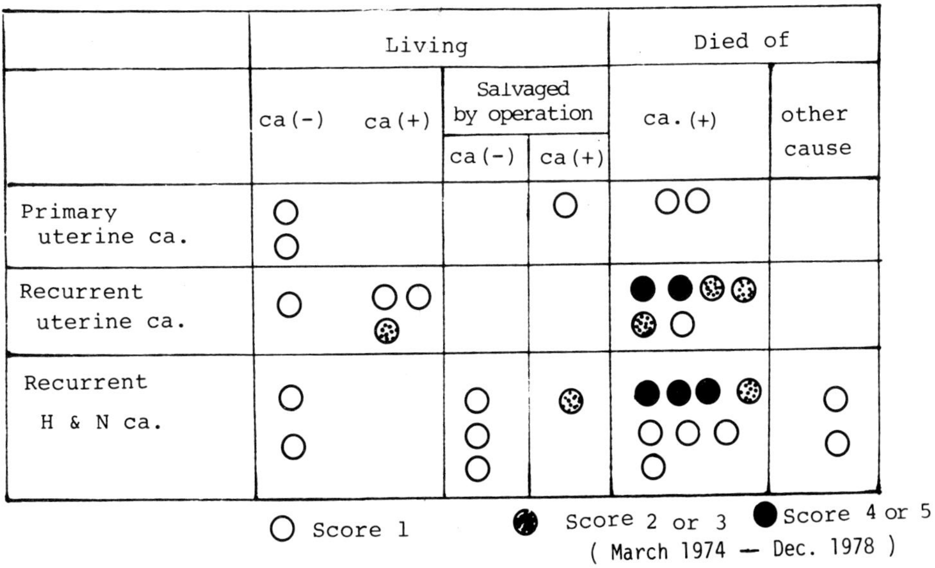

	Living		Salvaged by operation		Died of	
	ca(-)	ca(+)	ca(-)	ca(+)	ca.(+)	other cause
Primary uterine ca.	○ ○			○	○○	
Recurrent uterine ca.	○	○○ ⊛			●●⊛⊛ ⊛○	
Recurrent H & N ca.	○ ○		○ ○ ○	⊛	●●● ⊛ ○○○ ○	○ ○

○ Score 1   ⊛ Score 2 or 3   ● Score 4 or 5
(March 1974 — Dec. 1978)

Fig.9. Relationship between survival and early tumor effect score according to 3 groups of disease

112

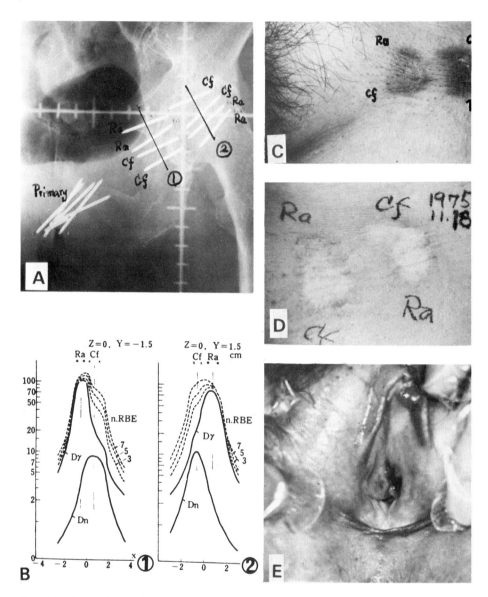

Fig. 10. Case 13. Primary malignant melanoma of the vagina, T1N0M0.
A: Implantation of Cf-252 needles was made in the primary site(E). Implantation of Ra and Cf-252 needles was made in the left inguinal region in the
   reversed order given as shown in (1) and (2) in A.
B: Dose rate curves along lines (1) and (2). The dotted lines(in this figure)
   represent the biological dose rates (D_n x RBE + D_γ) with assumed RBE
   values of n of 3, 5 and 7, respectively.
C,D:Early and late skin reactions over Ra and Cf-252 was almost identical indicating that the RBE value of n is estimated to be 5 - 7.

SUMMARY

This raport summarizes our clinical experience at the Cancer Institute Hospital from March 1974 to December 1978 with the use of small sources of Californium-252 on 65 cases consisting of 20 primary and 45 secondary cases. Radioresistant tumors of recurrent tumors developing from irradiated and/or operated scars were submitted to this therapy. Cf-252 needles, seeds and tubes were used as implants, surface molds and intracavitary application for various sites and conditions, either singly or combined with X-ray or Co-60 γ-rays. The results can be summarized as follows:

1. Good local control corresponding to score value of 1 was achieved in 30 out of 60 cases, which indicates that further continued clinical trial will be encouraging.

2. Most cases of head and neck cancer, skin cancer, malignant melanoma, papillary adenocarcinoma of the uterine cervix cancer have responded favorably to neutron dose of over 600 rad. On the contrary, carcinoma of the esophagus responded poorly to intracavitary boost therapy. This will need further clinical investigation.

3. No severe side effect except one case has been observed so far, suggesting a higher therapeutic advantage than Ra.

4. Preliminary clinical experience with Cf-252 seed assemblies on 12 cases was reported.

ACKNOWLEDGEMENT

This is to gratefully acknowledge that this work was supported in part by the U.S. Energy Research and Development Administration under Contract EY-76-C-09-0739 and Grants-in-Aid for Cancer Research from the Ministry of Education, Science and Culture and from the Ministry of Health and Welfare, Japan.

REFERENCES

1. Californium-252 Progress Report, No.20, 19-23, Jan. 1976.

2. Tsuya, A. et al. (1977) Nippon Acta Radio, 37, 238-247.

3. Tsuya, A. et al. (1979) Nippon Acta Radiol., 39, 643-653.

4. Onai, Y. et al. (1978) Nippon Acta Radiol. 38, 643-653.

5. Castro, J.R. et al. (1973) Am. J. Roentg. 117, 182-194.

6. Seydel, G.H. and Castro, J.V. (1975) Presented at the High LET Radiation Therapy Planning Seminar under the US-Japan Cooperative Cancer Research Program, Tokyo.

7. Vallejo, A. et al (1976) Int. J. Radiat. Oncol. Suppl. 1, 104.

114

8. Berry, R. et al. (1975) Afterloading: 20 years of experience, Proceeding of the Second International Symposium on Radiation Therapy, Memorial Sloan-Kettering Cancer Center, New York pp. 165-172.

9. Maruyama, Y. et al. (1978) Oncology 35, 172-178.

© 1979, Elsevier/North-Holland Biomedical Press
Treatment of Radioresistant Cancers
M. Abe, K. Sakamoto and T.L. Phillips eds.

RESULTS OF CLINICAL TRIAL WITH 30 MeV d-Be NEUTRONS AT NIRS

HIROSHI TSUNEMOTO, M.D., SHINROKU MORITA, M.D., TATSUO ARAI, M.D.

YUZURU KUTSUTANI, Ph.D., AKIRA KURISU, M.D. and YOICHIRO UMEGAKI, M.D.

National Institute of Radiological Sciences, 4-9-1, Anagawa, Chiba-City,

Chiba, Japan

INTRODUCTION

There are malignant tumors to be difficult to control, even though surgery or chemotherapy was effectively combined to radiation therapy.   One of these is the locally advanced tumor, in which the tumor lethal dose would be difficult to applied, because of a limit of tolerance dose of the normal tissues. And the other disease is radioresistant tumor , such as malignant melanoma, osteosarcoma or soft tissue sarcoma.

Recent radiobiological experiments suggest that the cells, distributed close to the necrotic area of tumor tissue were hypoxic and resistant to low LET radiations.   One the other hand, the radioresistant feature of the tumor cells might be explained by the wide shoulder of the dose cell survival curve obtained by irradiated cells.

In this report, a preliminary result of clinical trial with fast neutrons carring out at the hospital of National Institute of Radiological Sciences (NIRS), Chiba, Japan, is presented.   The purpose of this trial has been concentrated to examine the effect of high LET radiations, which charactarized by low OER and low repair capability of the irradiated cells.

METHOD OF TRIAL

(1) Charactaristics of the beam :

Fast neutron beam, obtained by bombarding a thick Beryllium target with 30 MeV deuterons, was used for clinical trial.   The dose rate was 45 rad/min. per 30 μA for 11.4 x 11.4 cm. field at STD 200 cm.   Contamination of gammer rays was less than 4 per cent.

(2) Treatment schedule:

Three types of schedule were used for this clinical trial (Table 1).

TABLE 1

TREATMENT SCHEDULE FOR FAST NEUTRON THERAPY

I : FAST NEUTRON ONLY :

    A)   130 rad x 12 fractions / 4 weeks

    B)   110 rad x 15 fractions / 5 weeks

    C)   90 rad x 18 fractions / 6 weeks

II : MIXED BEAM :

	Mon.	Tue.	Wed.	Thu.	Fri.
Radiation	N	X	X	X	N
Dose	72	170	170	170	72
	(5 weeks or 6 weeks)				

III : FAST NEUTRON BOOST :

    X - rays : 4000 - 5000 rad/4-5 weeks.

    Neutrons : 1500 rad x-ray equivalent dose

                in 1.5 - 2 weeks (shrinking field)

Fast neutron only was mainly applied in the treatment of radioresistant tumors, whereas mixed beam was used in the cases, in which the target volume to be irradiated has to be enlarged according to the extention of the tumor or critical organs were included unavoidably in the treatment volume.

TDF biologically equivalent concept was introduced as a method for estimation of the relationship between dose and effect (Nakamura, 1978)[1].

Response of the tumor and reactions of the normal tissues were recorded by applying a score system, for early reaction and late reaction, consisting of 5 steps.

Early reactions mean the reactions developing within 2 months after completion of therapy, while the reactions being manifest following 6 months were recorded as late reaction. An example of scores for early reaction is shown in Table 2.

TABLE 2

" EARLY EFFECT SCORES FOR EVALUATION OF FAST NEUTRON THERAPY "

    Tumor: 1) Disappear
            2) Regressing, less than half of original
            3) Regressing, larger than half size
            4) No shrinkage
            5) Growing

Skin reaction : 1) No change
                 2) Mild erythema
                 3) Marked erythema with or without dry
                    desquamation
                 4) Moist desquamation
                 5) Ulceration

Lung :   1) No change
                 2) Pneumonitis without clinical symptoms
                 3) Pneumonitis with slight clinical symptoms
                 4) Pneumonitis with severe clinical symptoms
                 5) Fetal pneumonitis

(3) Indication of clinical trial :

For carcinoma of the utrine cervix, a modified randomization study was used. The patients refered to the hospital during operation of the machine were participated to fast neutron therapy, whereas the patients were treated with x-rays, when the machine was in scheduled maintenance period.

(a) Carcinoma of the utrine cervix :

Five year survival rate of the patients suffering from carcinoma of the uterine cervix with over goose egg sized tumor, Staged T_3, was less than 50 per cent at NIRS hospital in radiation therapy which was clearly contrasted with the result for the patients with the tumor, smaller than goose egg sized.[2] Therefore, carcinoma of the uterine cervix, staged T_3 or T_{4a}, with over goose egg sized tumor was selected for this trial.

(b) Carcinoma of the lung :

The patients with carcinoma of the lung, staged T_1 or T_2, were participated for clinical trial, whereas the patients with obstructive pneumonia or pleural effsion were excluded. Pancoast' tumor was also included in this trial for improvement of local control or relief of syndrom.

(c) Carcinoma of the head & neck :

At the beginning of the study, carcinoma of the tongue staged T_3, N_{0-1}, M_0 was participated, because the rate of local control for those patients was less than 50 per cent.

However, it was difficult to estimate the effect of fast neutrons in the treatment of carcinoma of the tongue, because a interstitial irradiation has been combined with external radiation therapy in almost all cases. Therefore, the studies has been concentrated on the treatment of carcinoma of the pharynx, T_2 & T_3, and carcinoma of the larynx, T_3 & T_4.

(d) Carcinoma of the esophagus :

For carcinoma of the esophagus, the patients with the lesion less than 15 cm. long and with Karnofski index over 60 were candidated in this trial, while the patients with penetrated lesion were excluded.

(e) Carcinoma of the urinary organ :

The patients suffering from carcinoma of the urinary bladder and carcinoma of the prostate staged T_3 or T_4 (a part of the patients) were selected for the participants.

(f) Brain tumor :

Glioblastoma multiforme was the target for clinical trial. Fast neutron boost was applied.

(g) Carcinoma of the gastro-intestinal organ :

Fast neutron therapy was used as a curative modality for carcinoma of cardia of the stomach and carcinoma of the pancreatic gland. The reasons, why carcinoma of cardia of the stomach was selected as a target, could be explained by the fact that radiations would be considered as a radical therapy technique as same as surgery in this field.

(h) Radioresistant tumors :

Malignant melanoma, osteosarcoma and soft tissue sarcoma were selected for clinical trial with fast neutrons. Because the radioresistant feature of the malignant melanoma cells might be charactarized by the wide shoulder of dose cell survival curve of the irradiated cells, malignant melanoma was considered to be a typical target for high LET radiation therapy.

The patients with remote metastasis were excluded.

RESULT

Between November, 1975, and December, 1978, 397 patients have been treated with 30 MeV (d-Be) neutrons at NIRS (Table 3).

TABLE 3

NUMBER OF THE PATIENTS TREATED WITH 30 MeV(d-Be) NEUTRONS

AT NIRS (Nov. 1975 - Dec. 1978)

```
Female gynecological tumors ............. 112 ( 38 )
Carcinoma of the Esophagus .............. 46 (  3 )
Malignant Bone Tumor .................... 41 (  8 )
Carcinoma of the Head & Neck ........... 41 ( 15 )
Carcinoma of the Lung .................. 34 (  3 )
Malignant Melanoma ..................... 31 (  7 )
Soft Tissue Sarcoma .................... 20 (  6 )
Gioblastoma ............................ 11 (  0 )
Carcinoma of the Urinary Bladder ........ 9 (  1 )
Carcinoma of the Prostate .............. 9 (  0 )
Carcinoma of the Stomach ............... 7 (  0 )
Chordoma ............................... 6 (  6 )
Others ................................. 30 (  9 )
Total ................................. 397 ( 96 )
```

( ) : No. Patients with recurrent tumor.

As shown in this Table, female ginecological tumors were the largest number of the series, which followed by carcinoma of the esophagus, osteosarcoma and carcinoma of the head and neck.

The results evaluated according to early reaction score was summerized in Table 4.

Local control of the tumor was obtained in 41.4 per cent of the patients following fast neutron therapy, whereas complications have developed in only 8.4 per cent of this series. The reasons why the local control rate was low in the patients treated with fast neutron only might be explained by the fact that this schedule was mainly applied for the treatment of radioresistant tumors.

TABLE 4

LOCAL CONTROL RATE OF TUMOR AND RATE OF COMPLICATION FOLLOWING
FAST NEUTRON THERAPY (EARLY EFFECT)

	No of Patients	Local Control	Complication
Neutron Only	100	34 (34%)	15 (15%)
Mixed Beam	147	71 (48.2%)	8 (5.4%)
Neutron Boost	110	43 (39.1%)	7 (6.3%)
Total Cases	357	148 (41.4%)	30 (8.4%)

This analysis was carried out for 397 patients treated
between Nov., 1975 and December, 1978.
40 patients were excluded from this study; preoperative
irradiation 10, Bleeding of espphagus 1, others 29.

(a) Carcinoma of the utrine cervix :

The patients suffering from carcinoma of the uterine cervix have been treated with mixed beam of neutrons, which was a combination of whole pelvic irradiation, a dose equivalent to 5000 rad of x-rays, and a high dose rate intracavitary irradiation, 1000 - 1300 rad at the point A.

According to the results shown in Table 5, for medium sized tumor, local control rate for fast neutrons therapy was better than those treated with x-rays, whereas, for large tumor, no difference was observed in local control rate between the series of fast neutrons and x-rays. This results might suggest that, when the tumor size have become large enough beyond a limit, even fast neutrons, it seemed to be difficult to improve the results obtained by photon beams.

On the other hand, complications developed following fast neutron therapy were more marked than the series of x-rays.

TABLE 5

RESULTS OF CARCINOMA OF THE UTRINE CERVIX (STAGE III-B)

TREATED WITH FAST NEUTRONS (MIXED BEAM) OR PHOTON BEAM

SIZE OF TUMOR	LOCAL CONTROL		LOCAL FAILURE		COMPLICATION	
	NEUTRON	PHOTON	NEUTRON	PHOTON	NEUTRON	PHOTON
MEDIUM	10 / 12	15 / 21	2 / 12	6 / 21	3 / 12	3 / 21
	83.3#	71.4	16.0	28.5	25.0	14.2
LARGE	12 / 17	21 / 26	5 / 17	6 / 26	6 / 17	5 / 26
	70.5	80.7	29.4	23.1	25.2	19.2
	22 / 29	36 / 47	7 / 29	12 / 47	9 / 29	8 / 47
	76.8	76.5	24.1	25.5	31.0	17.0

: Per cent.   (Analized at March, 1979)

(b) Carcinoma of the lung :

Treatment results of surgery for carcinoma of the lung have been improved in recent years.   According to the report from National Cancer Center Hospital, 5 year survival rate of the patients with lung cancer was 30.1 per cent and 57.6 % for all patients and for Stage I respectively (Suemasu, 1979)[3]. On the other hand, results obtained by radiation therapy seemed to be not satisfactory in the present time, although almost all patients refered to this therapy were suffering from unresectable tumor.   However, it was suggested that radiations would be an effective and irreplaceable procedure for the cases with invasive tumor through chest wall or with some risk for surgery.

Table 6, which summerized the results of clinical trial with fast neutrons, shows that the local control rate was 5/9 and 2/2 when the estimation was carried out at 6 months and 24 months after completion therapy.

Relief of syndrom for the patients with Pancoast' tumor was excellent in fast neutron therapy.

TABLE 6

RESULTS OF CARCINOMA OF THE LUNG TREATED WITH 30 MeV(d-Be) NEUTRONS*

MONTHS OF SURVIVAL	3	6	9	12	18	24
SURVIVAL RATE	12/12	9/12	7/12	6/12	2/10	2/10
LOCAL CONTROL						
COMPLETE DISAPPEARANCE	4/12	5/9	5/7	2/6	2/2	2/2
INCOMPLETE DISAPPEARANCE	4/12	4/9	2/7	3/6	-	-
PARTIAL REGRESSION	4/12	-	-	1/6	-	-
COMPLICATION						
MODERATE FIBROSIS	6/12	5/9	4/7	2/6	1/1	1/1
SEVERE FIBROSIS	1/12	-	-	1/6	-	-

* : Adenocarcinoma & Squamous cell carcinoma.   (March, 1979)

(c) Carcinoma of the head and neck :

Results of fast neutron therapy is shown in Table 7. For carcinoma of the oral cavity, it was difficult to manage the huge tumor, invaded deeply into soft tissue.   It was suggested that combination of surgical procedures was recommended even for fast neutron therapy when the residual tumor was seen at the completion of radiation therapy.

The tumor arising from pharynx or larynx have been responded well to fast neutrons.

TABLE 7

PRELIMINARY RESULTS OF CARCINOMA OF THE HEAD & NECK
            TREATED WITH 30 MeV (d-Be) NEUTRONS (NIRS)

SITE	STAGE	LOCAL CONTROL	
TONGUE	T_3, N_{1-3}	3 / 8	
F. O. M.	T_3, N_{1-3}	1 / 4	
NASOPHARYNX	T_{3-4}, N_{0-2}	2 / 2	3 / 5
OROPHARYNX	T_3, N_{0-3}	1 / 3	
LARYNX	T_{3-4}, N_{0-2}	1 / 2	

(March, 1979)

122

(d) Carcinoma of the esophagus :

Of 14 patients received mixed beam or fast neutron boost, 9 (64 per cent) have been estimated as the local control.

A fast neutron dose equivalent to TDF 60 was necessary to obtaine the some pathological findings as those of x-rays in the surgical specimens.

(e) Carcinoma of the urinary organs :

8 patients with carcinoma of the prostate have been treated with fast neutron only.   All of the patients participated in this trial survived at December, 1978.   The tumor has responded well to fast neutrons and the surrounding tissues have well tolerated if the target volume was relatively small.

Carcinoma of the urinary bladder "T_3" has responded well to mixed beam or fast neutron boost, whereas the tumor "T_4" seemed to be not indicated for fast neutron therapy, because complications during or following therapy were severe and management of the patients was troublesome.

(f) Brain tumor :

The patients suffering from glioblastoma multiforme have been treated with fast neutron boost or mixed beam, in which the target volume has been reduced in size as much as possible.

TABLE 8

RESULT OF FAST NEUTRON THERAPY FOR GLIOBLASTOMA MULTIFORME (NIRS)

CODE	SEX	AGE	RT	SCORE	0 6 12 18 24 30 Months
50897	Female	16	M	II - II	II
51087	Male	51	B	II - IV	
51341	Male	27	M	II - II	II
51234	Male	32	B	II - IV	IV
51146	Male	22	M	II - II	II
51601	Female	64	M	II - III	
51934	Female	50	M	III - III	III
52065	Female	48	M	III - III	
52264	Female	51	M	III - IV	IV
52469	Male	61	M	II - II	II

M : Mixed Beam.   B : Neutron Boost.   (December, 1978)

The results of this series is shown in Table 8.   Mean survival time was 16 months.   16 year old female patient survived over 30 months and spent her active life.

(g) Carcinoma of the gastro-intestinal organs :

It was suggested in this trial that a dose equivalent to TDF 110 was necessary to control carcinoma of caria of the stomach and the pancreas, although a conclusion could not be obtained because of small number of participants.

(h) Osteosarcoma :

Local infusion of chemotherapeutic agents, such as Adriamycine etc., through regional artery followed by fast neutron only was the treatment choice of this trial.   After completion of radiation therapy, a systemic chemotherapy has been applied at the regular intervals for prevention of remote metastasis.

Table 9 shows the results obtained by examination of histopathological feature of the spesimens coming from the open biopsy or amputation.   There was no viable tumor cells following fast neutron therapy in 16 of 19 patients.

TABLE 9

LOCAL CONTROL OF OSTEOSARCOMA FOLLOWING FAST NEUTRON THERAPY,
ACCORDING TO HISTOLOGICAL EXAMINATION (NIRS)

| | NO. | TUMOR CELL | | CONTROL |
	PATIENTS	NEGATIVE	POSITIVE	RATE
OSTEOSARCOMA	17	15	2	15 / 17
CHONDROSARCOMA	2	1	1	1 / 2
TOTAL	19	16	3	16 / 19

(March, 1979)

As shown in Table 10, survival rate of the patients treated with fast neutrons seems to be better than those obtained by another modality.   However, severe fibrosis of the subcutaneous tissue has developed in 6 patients after completion of the therapy.

Preliminary results suggest that a dose equivalent to TDF 120 would be the upper limit of irradiation to avoid the severe late reaction.

An experiment carrying out with a transplantable human osteosarcoma cells in the nude mice suggested that RBE value of fast neutrons relative to 6 MV x-rays would be higher than 5.0 (Tatezaki, S.)[4].

124

TABLE 10

SURVIVAL CURVES FOR OSTEOSARCOMA TREATED WITH VARIOUS
MODALITIES

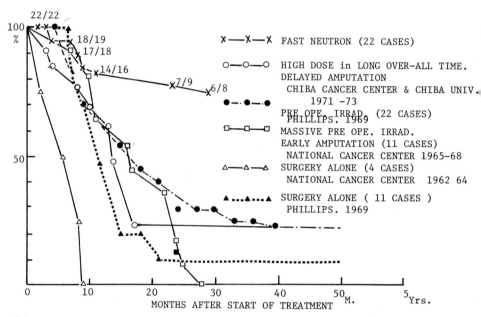

(i) Malignant melanoma :

   Malignant melanoma has responded well to fast neutrons (Table 11)

   However, survival rate of the patients suffering from malignant melanoma was
strongly depend on the presence or absence of metastasis into the regional
lymph nodes.   When the regional lymph nodes had been already effected at the
beginning of therapy, no patients might survive over 2 years.   For improvement
of this survival rate, various modalities have to be combined for the patients
with malignant melanoma, according to the stage of the disease.

TABLE 11

RESULTS OF MALIGNANT MELANOMA TREATED WITH 30 MeV (d-Be) NEUTRONS

MONTHS OF SURVIVAL	3	6	9	12	18	24	36
SURVIVAL RATE	26/26	23/26	19/23	14/21	7/17	5/15	2/13
LOCAL CONTROL							
COMPLETE DISAPPEARANCE	14/26	15/23	14/19	12/14	6/7	4/5	2/2
INCOMPLETE DISAPPEARANCE	6/26	4/23	1/19	-	-	-	-
PARTIAL REGRESSION OR GROWING	6/26	4/23	4/19	2/14	1/7	1/5	-
COMPLICATION							
MODERATE (3)	8/26	3/23	2/19	2/14	1/7	-	-
SEVERE (4 or 5)	1/26	-	-	1/14	-	-	-

(March, 1979)

(J) Soft tissue sarcoma :

Of 11 patients with soft tissue sarcoma, 7 have been in local control
(Table 12).

On the other hand, radiation ulcer has developed two year after completion
of therapy in a patient suffering from fibrosarcoma of the thigh. This case
expressed us the late reaction in soft tissue following high LET radiations
would be severer than that of low LET radiations.

TABLE 12

RESULTS OF SOFT TISSUE SARCOMA TREATED WITH 30MeV (d-Be) NEUTRONS

MONTHS OF SURVIVAL	3	6	9	12	18	24	36
SURVIVAL RATE	12/12	11/11	10/11	9/10	5/8	3/8	-
LOCAL CONTROL							
COMPLETE DISAPPEARANCE	5/12	7/9	6/8	5/7	3/5	2/3	-
INCOMPLETE DISAPPEARANCE	6/12	2/9	2/8	2/7	1/5	1/3	
PARTIAL REGRESSION	1/12	-	-	-	1/5	-	-
AMPUTATION	-	2	-	-	-	-	-
COMPLICATION							
MODERATE (3)	7/12	3/9	3/8	3/7	2/5	2/3	-
SEVERE (4 or 5)	-	-	-	-	-	1/3	

(March, 1979)

CONCLUSION

Clinical trials with fast neutrons suggest that local control rate of the locally advanced tumor and also radioresistant tumor could be improved by radiation therapy, when high LET radiations were effectively and carefully applied, and that the dose higher than TDF 120 would bring forth severe radiation damage. Therefore, the tumors which are considered to be difficult to eradicate by radiation therapy only, even with fast neutrons, has to be removed surgically following radiation therapy if it is accessible.   On the other hand, it was suggested that improvement of the dose distributions would be indispensable to make the best use of high LET radiation therapy.

REFERENCES

1. Protocol of clinical trial with fast neutrons for carcinoma of the utrine cervix, NIRS, 1978.

2. Nakamura, Y.: Treatment planning method in the use of the TDF biological equivalent concept in fast neutron therapy, Nippon Acta Radiol., 38, 950-960, 1978.

3. Suemasu, K.: Survival in research lung cancer, The Saishin Igaku, 34, 783-785, 1979.

4. Tatezaki, S.: Systemic multi-modal treatment of osteosarcoma, with special reference to the role of fast neutron radiotherapy, in Press.

© 1979, Elsevier/North-Holland Biomedical Press
Treatment of Radioresistant Cancers
M. Abe, K. Sakamoto and T.L. Phillips eds.

PRE-CLINICAL STUDIES OF NEGATIVE PI-MESONS AT TRIUMF

L. D. SKARSGARD, R. M. HENKELMAN, G. K. Y. LAM, B. PALCIC, C. J. EAVES AND
A. ITO[1]
Batho Biomedical Facility, TRIUMF, University of British Columbia, Vancouver,
B. C. V6T 1W5 Canada.
British Columbia Cancer Research Centre, 601 West 10th Avenue, Vancouver,
B. C. V5Z 1L3 Canada.

INTRODUCTION

Negative pi-mesons (π^- or pions), like neutrons, are a secondary radiation produced by bombarding a target with a primary beam of high energy particles. At TRIUMF[2], as at LAMPF[3] and at SIN[4], primary beams of accelerated protons are used to bombard the π^- production target. Because the efficiency for the production of pi-mesons is relatively low, intense beams of protons are required. At TRIUMF, a large sector-focusing isochronous cyclotron is used to provide the proton beam. A plan view of the facility is shown in Fig. 1. One of the advantages of this facility is that up to 4 separate proton beams can be extracted simultaneously from the cyclotron, the energy and intensity of each being individually variable. At present, two beams are being used, one of which is guided to the T2 target area from which the biomedical π^- beam is obtained. A Beryllium production target is normally used to inter- cept the proton beam at T2 and the biomedical beam line (M8) guides the collected π^- particles into the patient irradiation area. Figure 2 shows the layout of the beam line, which receives pi-mesons at an angle of 30° above the direction of the proton beam. The solid angle from which π^- are collected is approximately 10 millisteradians. The beam line consists of nine electro- magnets: five quadrupoles, two sextupoles and two 45° bending magnets or dipoles. The overall length of the beam line has been kept to a minimum, 7.5 m, which reduces the fraction of π^- which decay in flight. Also, the small take-off angle of 30° yields larger fluxes of high energy π^-, for which production is enhanced at small angles from the proton beam.

---

[1]Cyclotron Unit, Institute of Medical Science, University of Tokyo, Shirokane dai, Minato-ku, Tokyo 108, Japan.
[2]TRIUMF - TRI-University Meson Facility - Vancouver, B. C. Canada.
[3]LAMPF - Los Alamos Meson Physics Facility, Los Alamos, New Mexico, U. S. A.
[4]SIN - Schweitzischer Institut fur Nuklearforschung, Villigen, Switzerland.

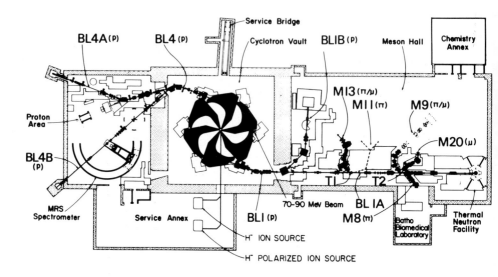

Fig. 1 Layout of TRIUMF. Existing beam lines are shown by solid lines, future installations by dashed lines. The biomedical beam line is the one designated M8, which delivers a horizontal beam into the patient treatment area.

The beam line was commissioned in 1975 and since that time a variety of pre-clinical studies have been carried out. Results of some of these studies have already been described[1-13]. These investigations include physical and dosimetric measurements as well as radiobiological experiments, using both *in vitro* and *in vivo* systems. The purpose of this paper is to present a brief review of the results of the pre-clinical program to date.

The dose rates at TRIUMF have been limited by the proton beam intensities available from the cyclotron, and this has hampered progress toward clinical use of the pi-meson beam. During 1978 and '79, proton currents of 100 μA have provided dose rates of 15 rads per minute to limited volumes and this has allowed us to begin studies of the effects of π^- beams on mouse and pig skin. Late in 1979, the first series of human skin nodule treatments will commence.

PHYSICAL MEASUREMENTS

A wide range of physical measurements has been made using the biomedical beam at TRIUMF to determine basic physical parameters of pion production and pion interactions in matter, to determine the optimal tuning of the biomedical channel, and to determine pion doses, dose distributions and microdosimetry of the various beams that have been developed for biological and medical

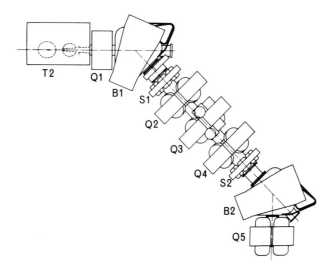

Fig. 2 Schematic of the biomedical beam line and the T2 meson production
        target.

irradiations.

The yields of negative particles have been measured as a function of the
mean channel momentum. Particle type has been determined by time-of-flight
techniques[5]. Results of such measurements for particles from a Carbon
target are shown in Fig. 3. The yield of mesons (π^- and μ^-, of which the
major component is π^-) increases sharply with increasing momentum, while the
electron yield decreases with increasing momentum. Furthermore, the yield of
electrons depends significantly on the distance from the point of production
of the pions to the exit face of the target. For the biomedical channel at
TRIUMF, particles are collected from the top surface of the target so that
if the proton beam is producing secondary particles near the top of the
target, fewer electrons result than if the production is near the bottom of
the target as shown in Fig. 3. Both the shape of the electron yield curve
and its dependence on the proximity of the point of production to the exit
face have been quantitatively explained with calculations which assume that
the electrons result from pair production by γ-rays from the decay of neutral
pions[13]. These studies have demonstrated that the channel must be operated
at high momentum ($\sim$180 MeV/c) and with minimal material between the production
point in the target and the exit face in order to ensure an acceptably low
electron contamination of the pion beam.

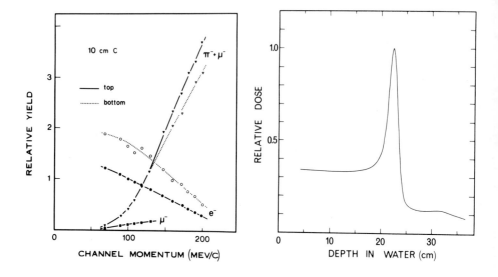

Fig. 3 Relative yield of particles from the biomedical beam line vs. particle momentum. The solid and dashed lines are the yields obtained when the proton beam is steered to the top or the bottom of the production target (10 cm of carbon), respectively.

Fig. 4 Depth dose profiles in water for a π^- beam of momentum 180 ± 3.8 MeV/c. The energy slit opening for this beam was 2.5 cm. μ^- and e^- account for the dose beyond the π^- peak, a small μ^- peak being evident at 31 cm.

One of the criteria for the tuning of the channel is to ensure that at the point where the pions of different momentum are spatially dispersed (at Q3, Fig. 2), there is minimal overlap of the different momenta[8]. This ensures that a narrow slit situated at this point will stop all but a monoenergetic beam of pions which will have a closely defined range. A depth dose curve for a narrow momentum beam is shown in Fig. 4. This curve was measured using a tissue equivalent plastic (Shonka A150) parallel plate ionization chamber with 1 mm gap and 20 mm diameter, filled with tissue equivalent gas. The ordinate is the measured charge without any corrections for ion chamber response. Because the pions were nearly monoenergetic (momentum = 180 ± 3.8 MeV/c), they stopped at a depth of 22.3 cm and deposited their star dose in a well defined peak with a peak to plateau dose ratio of 3. The width of the peak at 50% of the maximum dose was 3.0 cm. The tail beyond 25 cm depth is due to contaminant muons and electrons. Such a depth dose distribution dramatically illustrates the dose localization potential of pions, resulting from the process of star formation[3]. However, as the peak is spread to cover an extended volume, the peak to plateau ratio is reduced.

Because the radiation from pion stars is predominantly high LET, in
contrast to the low LET radiation from passing pions, dose alone is not an
adequate specification of the radiation for the interpretation of biological
effects. One method for obtaining a more detailed picture of the physical
character of the radiation is the measurement of microdosimetric spectra[14]
using a proportional counter[15]. Two such spectra are shown in Fig. 5.
These were measured in the plateau at a depth of 14.7 cm and in the peak at a

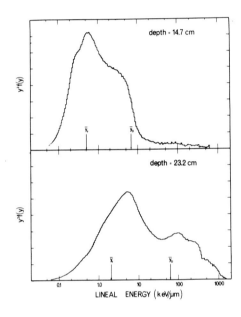

Fig. 5 Microdosimetric spectra
measured in the plateau (14.7 cm)
and peak (23.2 cm) regions of a
180 MeV/c π^- beam. The fractional
dose distribution, $Y^2f(Y)$ is
plotted vs. lineal energy, Y,
for both positions. $\bar{Y}_F$ and $\bar{Y}_D$
denote the mean lineal energies
averaged over frequency and
dose, respectively.

depth of 23.2 cm, using the beam for which the depth dose distribution is
shown in Fig. 4. It can be seen that in the plateau most of the events have
lineal energies below 10 keV/µm, whereas in the peak a large fraction of the
events are above 10 keV/µm. In the peak spectrum, the cut-off edges for
protons at 153 keV/µm and alpha particles at 432 keV/µm are clearly visible.
There are also significant numbers of events due to particles that are more
densely ionizing than α particles, above 500 keV/µm. The two conventional
averages[16], the frequency averaged lineal energy $\bar{y}_F$ and the dose averaged
lineal energy $\bar{y}_D$, are shown in Fig. 5 and are markedly different.

BIOLOGICAL MEASUREMENTS *IN VITRO*

The proportion of dose arising from high LET components thus varies considerably along the axis of a π⁻ beam, reaching a maximum at the distal side of the peak region. Consequently, it is to be expected that the radiobiological properties of the beam will vary with position in the π⁻ dose distribution, and detailed measurements are required to define these properties. In order to facilitate such studies, we developed a technique whereby mammalian cells are irradiated in a gelatin matrix[1, 3, 5 9].

Most of our *in vitro* measurements have been done using Chinese hamster (CHO) cells grown in spinner culture in MEM alpha medium (Flow Laboratories) supplemented with 10% Fetal calf serum. For π⁻ irradiations, cells were suspended in 37°C medium containing 25% gelatin (G8, Fisher Scientific) at a concentration of $2 - 5 \times 10^5$ cells/ml. This suspension was loaded into ABS (acrylonitrile butadiene styrene) plastic tubes, 1.2 cm inside diameter and 30 cm long, and cooled to 0°C. Each tube was then irradiated in a phantom which was also filled with 25% gelatin, as shown in Fig. 6.

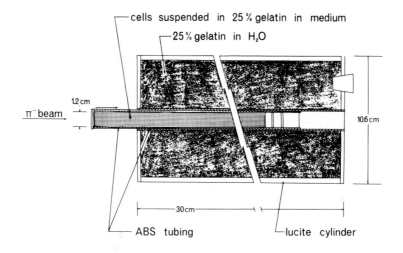

Fig. 6 Apparatus for irradiation of cells in 25% gelatin/medium. The sample tube was placed in a cylindrical phantom containing 25% gelatin and the entire unit was submerged in an ice-water tank and aligned with the π⁻ beam axis. In this illustration the sample tube is shown partially removed from the phantom. This arrangement provided as nearly as possible uniform attenuation for all particle paths, including those converging on the stopping region at relatively large angles from the axis of the π⁻ beam. Since the attenuation per cm of 25% gelatin is 1.08 times that of water[11] this is a significant consideration. ABS tubing (attenuation 1.03 x that of water) has replaced the polycarbonate

tubing (attenuation approx. 1.2 x that of water) used in our initial experiments because its attenuation more closely matches that of 25% gel/medium
and thus there is less perturbation of the particle paths.

The entire phantom was submerged in a large water tank, maintained at
$0^{\circ}C$, and the axis of the sample tube was aligned with the axis of the π^-
beam. After irradiation, the sample tube was removed from the phantom, the
gel was extruded from the tube and sliced at intervals of 2 mm or greater.
The slices were dissolved in $37^{\circ}C$ medium and appropriate aliquots were plated
in 5 cm plastic petri dishes. Colonies were stained and counted 8 days later.
Dosimetry for both x-rays (270 KVP, HVL 1.5 mm Cu) and π^- was based on
calibrations using Spokas tissue equivalent ionization chambers (0.1 and 0.5
cm^3).

This technique offers a number of advantages for studies such as this where
the radiobiological effect is to be mapped throughout a dose distribution: it
provides accurate, high resolution determination of the biological effect
throughout the volume because spatial positions can be accurately defined;

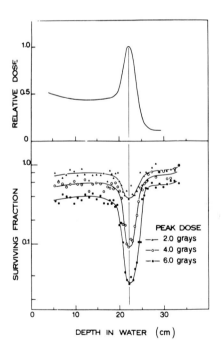

Fig. 7 Dose and cell survival
profiles for a narrow peak,
unmodulated π^- beam, 180 MeV/c
($FW_{0.8}$ = 2.5 cm). Survival of
CHO cells was measured in 25%
gelatin/medium at $0^{\circ}C$ with a
π^- dose rate of 12 rad/min.

the 25% gel/medium mixture has an elemental composition which is tissue
equivalent; at $0^{\circ}C$ there is no detectable dose-rate effect. The method has

been used to determine the Relative Biological Effectiveness (RBE) of π^- beams as a function of depth along the beam axis.

Figure 7 shows the results of an experiment in which a π^- beam of narrow momentum spread was used to irradiate three successive gel tubes with peak doses of 2, 4 or 6 grays. The momentum aperture in our beam line for this experiment was fixed at 3 cm, giving a relatively monoenergetic beam of momentum 180 MeV/c. The resulting depth dose profile (upper frame) shows a sharp peak at the end of the π^- range. The effect of this is seen in the survival profiles (lower frame) which show a sharp drop at the position of the dose maximum, illustrating the good spatial resolution of the gel system. It can be seen, from the line which has been drawn to bisect the dose peak, that there is some asymmetry between the dose and survival profiles in the peak region in this figure. Survival values on the downstream side of the peak are clearly depressed somewhat as a result of the increased RBE of the dose distribution in this region where star formation constitutes a larger fraction of the dose.

Cross-plots of survival profiles such as those shown in Fig. 7 provide survival vs. dose responses from which RBE values can be determined and compared to conventional X-ray responses. Table I shows RBE values for 50% survival at various positions along the axis of the π^- beam illustrated in Fig. 7. As expected, the RBE increases with depth in the stopping region. In the entrance or plateau region, the RBE relative to 270 KVP X-rays is not significantly different from 1.0.

TABLE I

RBE VALUES : π^- NARROW PEAK

POSITION	DEPTH	*$RBE_{0.5}$
X-rays	–	1.0
Plateau	5-18 cm	1.0
Upstream	20.5 cm	1.15
Peak center	22.0 cm	1.3
Downstream	23.5 cm	1.6

*uncertainties in these preliminary RBE values are approximately ±20%.

For radiotherapy applications the peak must be extended over a larger depth range by modulation of the energy of the pions. This can be

accomplished at TRIUMF by dynamic adjustment of the momentum defining slits
in the beam line. Figure 8 (upper frame) shows the depth dose profile for
such a beam, modulated so as to give a uniform dose over the depth range
from 19 to 26 cm. The peak width is 7.5 cm when measured at 90% of maximum

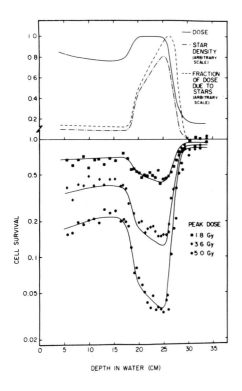

Fig. 8 Dose and cell survival
profiles for a modulated π^-
beam – 7 cm peak. π^- momentum
180 ± 12 MeV/c. Upper frame
shows relative dose, star density
and star dose fraction profiles
along π^- beam axis. Lower frame:
data points are measured survival
values for CHO cells in 25%
gelatin/medium for three different
peak doses; solid curves are
fitted responses calculated from
Eq (1).

dose. This beam tune was generated by the beam line control computer, using
a linear programming technique[7]. With this technique a dose distribution
of specified properties is generated from a number of appropriate static
momentum distributions. It can be optimized to provide maximum dose rate
(as in the case shown) or minimum entrance dose. Although this particular
distribution was specified to be flat to within ±1% in the peak region in
order to facilitate a study of variations in RBE through the stopping region,
any desired peak shape can be generated by this method.

In the lower half of Fig. 8 are shown the corresponding cell survival
profiles for three different gel tubes, each receiving a different peak dose.
It can be seen that in the peak region, although the dose is uniform, cell

survival decreases with increasing depth, again reflecting an increase in RBE toward the distal side of the peak where the star contribution is greatest. Similar depth effects have been reported by Raju et al.[17]. The variation in the star contribution with depth is illustrated by the measured star density and the fraction of dose due to stars, both of which are plotted in the upper frame of Fig. 8. The relative star density was obtained from particle stopping distributions measured with a small scintillator telescope.

In an attempt to relate the biological effectiveness to the radiation qualtiy at different positions in the π^- dose distribution, the survival data of Fig. 8 were fitted with a cell survival model in which the star fraction is used to characterize the physical properites of the beam. If one assumes that star events will influence primarily single-event killing, then applying the linear-quadratic model of inactivation, cell survival can be expressed as

$$S = \exp(-C_1 D - C_2 f_s D - C_3 D^2) \qquad (1)$$

where f_s is proportional to the fraction of dose from stars

C_1 is the inactivation constant for non-star single events

C_2 is the inactivation constant for star single events and its value is coupled to f_s

C_3 is the inactivation constant for two-event inactivation

S is the surviving fraction and D is the total dose.

Fitting equation (1) to the data of Fig. 8 gives values for C_1, C_2 and C_3 of 0.13 ± 0.02 gray^{-1}, 0.24 ± 0.02 gray^{-1} and 0.064 ± 0.005 gray^{-2}, respectively. The solid lines in the lower portion of Fig. 8 represent the fitted survival profiles (reference 10 provides more details of this method).

Once the parameters of this model have been determined, the model can be used to calculate a number of relevant properties of the beam, such as the survival vs. dose response for any depth along the π^- beam axis[18] or the RBE vs. depth response for any given dose or survival level. Figure 9 shows such calculated RBE vs. depth responses for the beam represented in Fig. 8. The RBE values shown in Fig. 9 have been normalized to a value of 1.0 in the plateau region at a depth of 15 cm, and they have been calculated for several different survival levels. It is evident that the RBE reaches a maximum at, or just beyond the distal edge of the extended peak.

This model, therefore, allows more efficient use of the radiobiological measurements made at different positions in a given π^- dose distribution. It also offers the possibility of predicting the biological properties of new

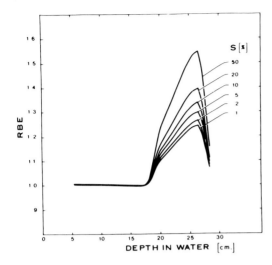

Fig. 9 RBE as a function of depth, calculated from Eq (1) for various survival levels (S = 0.01 to 0.5). RBE values are normalized to a value of 1.0 in the plateau, depth 15.0 cm.

dose distributions from measurements of the star density along the beam axis. This may be of significant value in treatment planning, when new beam tunes are required for particular clinical situations.

Table II shows a summary of RBE values measured *in vitro* at TRIUMF, as well as some representative values from LAMPF and SIN (for a more complete review see reference (19)). RBE values are tabulated for both the center of the stopping peak and for the plateau (on the proximal side of the peak), where available. Values of the Oxygen Gain Factor (OGF) are also compared in this rable. It is defined as

$$OGF = (OER)_s / (OER)_\pi$$

where $(OER)_s$ is the oxygen enhancement ratio measured for the specified "conventional" radiation, and $(OER)_\pi$ is the value for the stopping peak region. Beam characteristics (dose rate, width of stopping peak measured at 80% of maximum – $FW_{0.8}$) are given in column 2. Except as noted, the studies have used unmodulated beams. The low dose rates available for many of the experiments required precautions to minimize dose rate effects. At TRIUMF this was accomplished by irradiating at 0°C.

OER determinations at TRIUMF have been made using the following procedure: CHO cells were suspended in 25% gelatin/medium and 0.5 ml samples were loaded into 6 ml glass tubes. For aerobic irradiations the cell concentration was 2×10^5 cells/ml and the tubes were stored and irradiated at 0°C without

TABLE II

RBE AND OGF VALUES FOR CULTURED CELL SURVIVAL

CELL LINE	BEAM	COMPARISON RADIATION	PLATEAU RBE	PEAK RBE	OGF	COMMENTS	REFERENCE
CHINESE HAMSTER CELLS CH2B2	TRIUMF (2 RAD/MIN) $FW_{0.8}$ = 6 CM	^{60}Co	1.0	1.5	-	AT S = 0.1	(3) SKARSGARD ET AL. (1977)
CHINESE HAMSTER CELLS CHO	TRIUMF (12 RAD/MIN) $FW_{0.8}$ = 2.5 CM	270 KVP	1.0	1.3	-	AT S = 0.5	THIS REPORT
CHINESE HAMSTER CELLS CHO	TRIUMF (25 RAD/MIN) $FW_{0.8}$ = 6 CM	270 KVP	-	1.3	1.2	AT S = 0.1	(20) PALCIC & SKARSGARD (1979)
CHINESE HAMSTER CELLS CHO	TRIUMF (10 RAD/MIN) MODULATED - 7 CM	270 KVP	1.0	1.3 1.2	- -	AT S = 0.5 AT S = 0.1	THIS REPORT
MOUSE L5178Y CELLS	TRIUMF (2 RAD/MIN) $FW_{0.8}$ = 6 CM	^{60}Co	1.0	1.4	-	AT S = 0.5	(21) OKADA ET AL. (1979)
HUMAN KIDNEY CELLS T1	LAMPF (5 RAD/MIN) $FW_{0.8}$ = 2 CM	-- PLATEAU	-	2.0	-	AT S = 0.5	(22) RAJU ET AL. (1975)
HUMAN KIDNEY CELLS T1	LAMPF (5 RAD/MIN) $FW_{0.8}$ = 4.5 CM	250 KVP	-	1.4	-	AT S = 0.4	(23) TODD ET AL. (1975)
CHINESE HAMSTER CELLS V79	LAMPF (25 RAD/MIN) $FW_{0.8}$ = 2 CM	250 KVP	-	1.6-1.7	1.3	AT S = 0.1-0.5	(24) RAJU ET AL. (1979)
HUMAN KIDNEY CELLS T1	LAMPF (10 RAD/MIN) MODULATED - 10 CM	^{60}Co	-	1.5	-	AT S = 0.5	(25) RAJU ET AL. (1978)
CHINESE HAMSTER CELLS V79	LAMPF (10 RAD/MIN) MODULATED - 5 CM -10 CM	250 KVP 250 KVP	1.0 -	1.4-1.6 1.1	1.2 1.3	AT S = 0.1-0.5 AT S = 0.1-0.5	(24) RAJU ET AL. (1979)
CHINESE HAMSTER CELLS V79	LAMPF (10 RAD/MIN) MODULATED - 10 CM	^{60}Co	-	-	1.7	AT S = 0.1	(26) HALL & ASTOR (1979)
CHINESE HAMSTER CELLS V79	SIN (4 RAD/MIN) $FW_{0.8}$ = 4 CM	^{60}Co	1.1	1.8	-	AT S = 0.1	(27) DERTINGER ET AL. (1976)
CHINESE HAMSTER CELLS 19/1	SIN (6 RAD/MIN) $FW_{0.8}$ = 4 CM	140 KVP	0.8-1.0	1.3	-	AT S = 0.5-0.1	(28) TREMP ET AL. (1979)

gassing. For hypoxic samples the cell concentration was 2×10^6 cells/ml and the tubes were gassed with N_2 during 2 hours incubation at 37°C, cooled to 0°C, and a 4 ml overlay of deoxygenated phosphate buffered saline was added to each tube. This overlay was bubbled with N_2 for an additional 1 hr. at 0°C before the tubes were sealed and irradiated at 0°C.

The data in Table II show quite good consistency, generally, between the three facilities, considering the different cell lines and techniques used. Plateau RBE values are very close to 1.0, while peak values range from 1.3 to 2.0 for unmodulated beams and from 1.1 to 1.6 for modulated beams, when measured for surviving fractions of S = 0.1 to 0.5. OGF values at both TRIUMF and LAMPF are in close agreement (1.2 - 1.3) except for the Hall and Astor[26] measurement of 1.7, which may be the result of an anomalously high OER of 3.8 for ^{60}Co.

All of the data shown in Table II pertain to experiments where the doses have been delivered in single fractions.

Other *in vitro* studies carried out at TRIUMF include measurements of split-dose recovery and determinations of the yield of DNA strand breaks. Recovery between divided doses of both peak and plateau pions appears to be comparable to the levels of recovery observed between divided X-ray doses, for recovery periods of up to 4 hours. This is consistent with results of Todd et al.[23] and Mill et al.[29]. The RBE for the production of DNA strand breaks was 0.7, as would be expected if most of these are the result of a single primary event[30]. Similar results were obtained at SIN by Weibezahn et al.[31] and at TRIUMF by Okada[21], who also measured mutation induction in mouse L5178Y cells.

BIOLOGICAL MEASUREMENTS *IN VIVO*

Preliminary estimates of the RBE values for stem cell populations in two different normal tissues, marrow and skin, have now been obtained from experiments carried out at TRIUMF.

The response of marrow was measured using two endpoints: spleen colony formation *in vivo*[32], and granulocyte/monocyte/macrophage colony formation *in vitro*[33, 34]. These endpoints detect two different, although closely related, stem cell populations[35]. Cells that generate macroscopic spleen colonies in lethally irradiated syngeneic recipient mice are operationally referred to as CFU-S and have been shown to be both pluripotent and capable of extensive self-renewal. Cells detected by their ability to produce granulopoietic colonies *in vitro* are operationally referred to as CFU-C. These represent a derivative population with restricted differentiation and proliferative potential. Together CFU-S and CFU-C comprise less than 1% of the total marrow population.

In the present experiments femoral marrow cells were removed from (C57B1/6B x C3H/HeB)F$_1$ mice and suspended in 25% gelatin[3] for irradiation. For π^- irradiations the same set-up and beam tune were used as described above for OER measurements on CHO cells but gassing with either N$_2$ or O$_2$ was omitted. In each experiment aliquots of the same marrow cell-gelatin mix were irradiated with 270 KVP X-rays. All cells were kept on ice until assayed. This served the dual purpose of minimizing potential dose rate effects inherent in the use of π^- dose rates of 2-3 rads/min, and of maintaining maximal CFU-S and CFU-C viability during the period (up to 8 hours) required to complete irradiations. CFU-S and CFU-C were then assayed by routine procedures[36,37].

RBE values for cells irradiated in the peak and plateau regions are given
in Table III. The results comparing π^- and X-ray effects on CFU-S and CFU-C
are similar, and appear to agree with those obtained using the Los Alamos
facility where a beam tune with a somewhat narrower peak was employed[38].

TABLE III

RBE VALUES FOR NORMAL TISSUES

TISSUE	ENDPOINT	π^- BEAM	COMPARISON RADIATION	PLATEAU RBE	PEAK RBE	COMMENTS	REFERENCE
BONE MARROW	CFU-S	TRIUMF (2-3 RADS/MIN)	270 KVP	1.0	1-1.1	s = 0.1-0.5	THIS REPORT
	CFU-S	LAMPF (4-6 RADS/MIN)	^{60}Co	~1.0	~1.0	s = 0.1-0.5	(38) CARLSON & THORNTON (1976)
	CFU-C	TRIUMF (2-3 RADS/MIN)	270 KVP ^{60}Co	0.8-1.0 1.1-1.3	1.0-1.1 1.4-1.5	s = 0.1-0.5 s = 0.1-0.5	THIS REPORT
SKIN	MOUSE FOOT ACUTE SKIN REACTION	TRIUMF (15 RADS/MIN)	270 KVP	- - -	1.1 1.2 1.4-1.6	1F 2F 10F	THIS REPORT
		LAMPF (80 RADS/MIN)	300 KVP	- - -	1.1 1.3 1.4	1F 2F 5F	(24) RAJU ET AL. (1979)
		SIN (30 RADS/MIN)	200 KVP	0.85	1.15-1.25	1F	(39) FRÖHLICH ET AL. (1979)

However, the reference radiation in their studies was a ^{60}Co γ-ray source.
Comparison of our π^- results with previous data using ^{60}Co γ-rays yields
higher RBE values (Table III).

The response of skin was evaluated using the mouse foot system as modified
in our laboratory[40]. Three experiments were performed and from these
preliminary estimates of the RBE for acute skin reactions have been obtained
(Table III). These include results for single doses (1F) as well as for 2
equal fractions (2F) spaced 24 hours apart and for 10 equal fractions (10F)
given at approximately 7 hour intervals (Fig. 10). For π^- irradiations,
mice were irradiated 3 at a time in a jig that allowed only one hind foot
from each mouse to be irradiated using appropriate collimation and a perspex
positioning apparatus. The design of this jig was adapted from that used
for matched X-ray irradiations. Mice were held unanaesthetized in the same
lead boxes[40] but these were stacked vertically rather than horizontally

with the protruding feet to be irradiated held in alignment with the axis
of the π⁻ beam by a modular, solid perspex mould. The jig was then positioned
such that the toe and heel of each foot was contained in a 2 cm length that
coincided with the peak of the beam (180 ± 12 MeV/c).

In each experiment parallel groups of mice were irradiated with 270 KVP
X-rays as previously described with a slight modification in the jig design
to match the π⁻ dose rate (which averaged 14-15 rads/min). During all
irradiations mice were gassed with pure O_2. RBE values were calculated from
curves fitted by eye to the 7 day average reactions (K_7's) obtained in π⁻
versus X-irradiated mice.

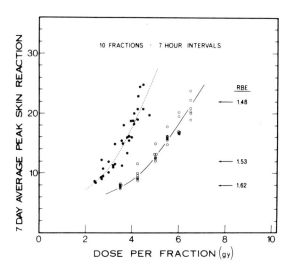

Fig. 10 Acute skin
reaction dose response
curves for mice given 10
equal fractions of π⁻
or 270 KVP X-rays. One
experiment: each point
represents an individual
animal, open circles –
X-rays, solid circles –
π⁻.

The results shown in Fig. 10 strongly support the view that the RBE for
acute skin reactions is dose dependent. This was anticipated from previous
results with neutrons[41] and the recent results of 1, 2 and 5 fraction
experiments obtained by Raju et al.[24] using the LAMPF π⁻ beam. It should
be noted that our RBE values obtained from the 1 and 2 fraction experiments
may prove to be in part a function of the low dose rate employed, and at
higher dose rates slightly lower RBE values might be expected. For 10
fractions (i.e. doses of 300-500 rads X-rays per fraction) a dose rate effect
(between 158 and 15 rads/min) has not been demonstrable[42] and the 10F RBE
value obtained at 15 rads/min is therefore unlikely to change as a result of
improved π⁻ dose rates. More experiments will, however, be required to
establish whether the RBE for acute skin reactions continues to increase

with increasing fraction number, i.e. decreasing dose per fraction and hence increasing survival per fraction. This will be of particular interest for future comparison of the RBE for normal tissue tolerance obtained during the course of clinical trials where somewhat higher fraction numbers and lower doses per fraction are likely to be employed.

CONCLUSIONS

Pre-clinical investigation of the π^- beam at TRIUMF has provided a considerable body of information on the physical and biological properties of this new radiation. The physical measurements have facilitated optimization of the quality and intensity of the π^- beam and have provided a sound basis for dosimetry measurements. *In vitro* biological studies with cultured cells have made it possible to accurately map the biological effectiveness of the beam throughout the dose distribution, and may permit prediction of the biological effectiveness of new beams from a simple physical characterization. *In vivo* studies using the mouse foot system have yielded RBE values for fractionated doses which are consistent with the early data from LAMPF for normal tissue effects in humans[43-45]. There is also quite good agreement between the results obtained from the pre-clinical programs at each of the three major π^- facilities, LAMPF, SIN and TRIUMF.

While many studies remain to be completed, particularly in the *in vivo* program, the pre-clinical investigations at TRIUMF have reached the point where the initiation of patient treatment can be contemplated. Irradiation of human skin tumour nodules will be the first such treatment and this is expected to begin in November, 1979.

ACKNOWLEDGEMENTS

The co-operation of the TRIUMF staff is gratefully acknowledged, as is the skillful technical assistance of R. W. Harrison, B. Jaggi, I. Harrison, N. McKinney, H. Adomat, C. Smith and J. Bragg. This work was supported by the British Columbia Cancer Foundation and the National Cancer Institute of Canada. One of the Authors (C. J. E.) is a Research Associate of the National Cancer Institute of Canada.

REFERENCES

1. Skarsgard, L. D. and Palcic, B. (1974) In: Proceedings of the XIIIth International Congress Series No. 399, Radiology, Vol. 2, pp. 447-454 Exerpta Medica, Amsterdam.

2. Henkelman, R. M. et al. (1977) Int. J. Radiat. Oncol. Biol. Phys., 2,

123-127.

3. Skarsgard, L. D. et al. (1977) In: Proceedings of the International Symposium on Radiobiological Research needed for the Improvement of Radiotherapy, IAEA, Vienna, Austria, Nov. 1976 Vol. 2, 87-100.

4. Lam, G. K. Y. et al. (1978) Phys. Med. Biol., 23, 768-776.

5. Henkelman, R. M. et al. (1977) TRIUMF External Report TRI-77-2.

6. Shortt, K. R. and Henkelman, R. M. (1978) Phys. Med. Biol., 23, 495-498.

7. Lam, G. K. Y. et al. (1978) Submitted to Phys. Med. Biol.

8. Henkelman, R. M. et al. (1978) Nucl. Instr. and Meth., 155, 317-324.

9. Skarsgard, L. D. et al. (1977) International Atomic Energy Agency, Advisory Group Meeting on Clinical Applications of Particle Radiation and the Role of Radiosensitivity Modifiers, Vienna, December 19-21 (in press).

10. Henkelman, R. M. and Lam, G. K. Y. (1978) In: Proceedings of 6th Symposium on Microdosimetry, Vol. I. Booz, J., Ebert, H. G. (eds), pp. 497-506.

11. Nordin, J. A. and Henkelman, R. M. (1979) Phys. Med. Biol. (in press).

12. Harrison, R. W. (1972) TRIUMF Report TRI-72-1.

13. Poon, M. N. (1977) M.Sc. Thesis, University of British Columbia.

14. Ito, A. and Henkelman, R. M. (1979) Submitted to Radiat. Res.

15. Rossi, H. H. and Rosenzweig, W. (1955) Radiology, 64, 404-411.

16. Kellerer, A. M. and Rossi, H. H. (1969) In: Proceedings of the Second Symposium on Microdosimetry, EUR 4452 d-e-f, pp. 843-853.

17. Raju, M. R. et al. (1978) Int. J. Radiat. Oncol. Biol. Phys., 4, 841-844.

18. Skarsgard, L. D. et al. (1979) Rad. & Environm. Biophys. (in press).

19. Skarsgard, L. D. (1979) In: Proceedings of the Sixth International Congress of Radiation Research (in press).

20. Palcic, B. and Skarsgard, L. D. (1979) Unpublished data.

21. Okada, S. (1979) Private communication.

22. Raju, M. R. et al. (1975) Radiology, 116, 191-193.

23. Todd, P. et al. (1975) Radiology, 116, 179-180.

24. Raju, M. R. et al. (1979) Brit. J. Radiol. (in press).

25. Raju, M. R. et al. (1978) Brit. J. Radiol., 51, 704-711.

26. Hall, E. J. and Astor, M. (1979) Int. J. Radiat. Oncol. Biol. Phys., 5, 55-60.

27. Dertinger, H. et al. (1976) Int. J. Radiat. Biol., 29, 271-277.

28. Tremp, J. et al. (1979) Rad. & Environm. Biophys. (in press).

29. Mill, A. J. et al. (1976) Brit. J. Radiol., 49, 357-359.

30. Palcic, B. and Skarsgard, L. D. (1978) Unpublished data.

31. Weibezahn, K. F. et al. (1979) Rad. & Environm. Biophys. (in press).

32. Till, J. E. and McCulloch, E. A. (1961) Radiat. Res., 14, 213-222.

33. Pluznik, D. H. and Sachs, L. (1965) J. Cell. Comp. Physiol., 66, 319-324.

34. Bradley, T. R. and Metcalf, D. (1966) Aust. J. Exp. Biol. Med. Sci., 44, 287-300.

35. McCulloch, E. A. and Till, J. E. (1971) Am. J. Pathol., 65, 601-619.

36. Humphries, R. K. et al. (1979) Blood, 53, 746-763.

37. Gregory, C. J. and Eaves, A. C. (1978) In: Differentiation of Normal and Neoplastic Hematopoietic Cells, pp. 179-192 (Clarkson, B., Marks, P. A. and Till, J. E. Eds).

38. Carlson, D. E. and Thornton, J. (1976) Radiol., 120, 213-215.

39. Fröhlich, E. M. et al. (1979) Rad. & Environm. Biophys. (in press).

40. Douglas, B. G. et al. (1979) Radiat. Res., 77, 453-471.

41. Field, S. B. and Hornsey, S. (1971) Europ. J. Cancer, 7, 161-169.

42. Eaves, C. J. (1978) Unpublished observations.

43. Kligerman, M. M. et al. (1976) Am. J. Radiol., 126, 261-267.

44. Kligerman, M. M. et al. (1977) Int. J. Radiat. Oncol. Biol. Phys., 3, 335-339.

45. Kligerman, M. M. et al. (1978) Int. J. Radiat. Oncol. Biol. Phys., 4, 263-265.

© 1979, Elsevier/North-Holland Biomedical Press
Treatment of Radioresistant Cancers
M. Abe, K. Sakamoto and T.L. Phillips eds.

CURRENT OBSERVATIONS OF PION RADIATION THERAPY AT LAMPF[1]

M. Kligerman,[2] H. Tsujii,[3] M. Bagshaw,[4] S. Wilson, W. C. Black III, F. Mettler, K. Hogstrom

Cancer Research and Treatment Center, University of New Mexico, Albuquerque, New Mexico USA 87131

ABSTRACT

Fifty-three of the ninety-three patients treated to-date have had peak pion doses of 2700 rads or more. This is the minimal dose which has resulted in longer-term complete disappearance of the tumor. These fifty-three patients have been followed for five to twenty-four months. They are separated into those who have received less than 3300 rads (the earlier cases) and those who received over 3300 rads. Most of the latter have only been observed since July 1978. Acute reactions have been modest with the lower doses. However, reactions have been increasing in number and severity with use of the higher dose levels. No serious late changes have been observed to date, although this could alter now that higher doses are used routinely. Considering that the patients selected for pion radiotherapy have advanced local cancer, responses have been encouraging.

Keywords: particle radiotherapy, high linear energy transfer (high LET), negative pi mesons (pions), clinical trials, therapeutic gain

---

[1] These investigations were supported in part by U.S. Public Health Service Grants No. CA-16127 and No. CA-14052 from the National Cancer Institute, Division of Research Resources and Centers, and by the U.S. Department of Energy.

[2] Cancer Research and Treatment Center, University of New Mexico, Albuquerque, New Mexico and the Los Alamos Scientific Laboratory, Los Alamos, New Mexico 87545

[3] Radiation Oncology Fellow. Permanent address: Hokkaido University, Sapporo, Japan

[4] Visiting Research Professor of Radiation Oncology. Permanent address: Stanford University, Palo Alto, California

INTRODUCTION

Phase I-II studies leading to randomized clinical trials of pion radiotherapy are nearing completion at the Clinton P. Anderson Meson Physics
Facility, Los Alamos, New Mexico. These studies are being conducted jointly by
the University of New Mexico Cancer Research and Treatment Center (UNM/CRTC),
Albuquerque, and the Los Alamos Scientific Laboratory (LASL). The objective
of these studies has been: (1) to establish tolerance of various normal tissues
to pions as compared to conventional radiotherapy; (2) to observe effects of
pions on tumor regression and regrowth; and (3) to determine initial dose
schedules for randomized clinical trials of pion radiotherapy.

As of April 15, 1979, a total of 93 patients had been treated or were
under treatment with pions at Los Alamos, all but four of them since June 1976.
Twenty of these patients have received additive conventional treatment to pion-
treated portals. Nine of the patients were in the initial series of tests on
patients with multiple tumor nodules in and below the skin, 74 (Table 1) had
advanced or recurrent primaries (one patient had two primaries histologically
distinguishable into a bladder carcinoma and a prostatic carcinoma), and 10
had miscellaneous metastases.

Each time a new anatomic structure was placed under treatment, the prescribed dose levels were kept low to avoid unexpected serious untoward effects.
Initial doses for each normal tissue site were decided by taking 60% of the
conventional radiotherapy curative dose and dividing it by a safety factor of
two. Subsequent doses were then slowly escalated as each dose level appeared
to be well tolerated. Studies began with the skin and then progressed to the
oral cavity, pharynx, and larynx; rectum and bladder; and finally lung and
abdominal structures. Initially, many of the patients treated had extremely
advanced lesions and many had existing distant metastases at the time of
treatment. When pion radiotherapy was well tolerated and it was not possible
because of accelerator schedules to add more pion treatment after minimal acute
reactions, additive conventional radiation was given. The amount of additive
conventional radiation that could be added was a measure of the tissue
tolerance to pions. However, seven patients were given additive conventional
radiation when a mechanical target failure precluded completion of their
treatment with pions. Surgery was also performed when it appeared it would be
beneficial and feasible. No problems have been encountered in adding conventional radiation or performing surgery on pion-treated patients. Those with
distant metastases were placed on chemotherapy when it was medically indicated.

TABLE 1

PRIMARIES TREATED WITH PIONS

Site	Total	Pions Alone	Pions Plus Conventional
Brain	9	8	1
Nasopharynx	5	4	1
Oropharynx	8	4	4
Hypopharynx	1	1	0
Larynx	4	1	3
Oral Cavity	4	4	0
Salivary Gland	1	0	1
Esophagus	1	1	0
Superior Sulcus	2	1	1
Lung	1	1	0
Breast*	1	0	1
Pancreas	15	14	1
Stomach	1	0	1
Prostate	9	8**	1
Liver	1	1	0
Urinary Bladder	2	2**	0
Colon	1	1	0
Rectum	6	4	2
Skin	2	1	1
Sarcoma	1	1	0
TOTAL	75	57	18

_____

*Male Breast

**One Patient, 2 Primaries

To obtain a relatively uniform biological effect across the modulated peak, those static beams having a peak depth (Z) dimension less than 8 cm have a flat total physical dose; whereas in those with a Z dimension of 9 cm to 14 cm, a respective gradient of approximately 10-40% from the proximal to distal portion of the peak is required. Therefore, opposed portals with stopping regions superimposed at depth are used in most patient treatments (laterals for head and neck, and anterior-posterior/posterior-anterior for other sites). This appears to provide relatively uniform dose and clinical-biological effect across the treatment volumes. The modulated peak dimension and the collimator are designed for individual portals to fit the physical peak dose distribution to the tumor treatment volumes (Hogstrom et al.)[1]

Since local control was not achieved in any patient treated with pions alone who received less than 2700 peak pion rads, this paper presents a pre-liminary assessment of those 53 patients who received a minimum of 2700 peak pion rads and who have been followed for at least five months and as long as 24 months. Acute reactions in patients treated by relatively low doses prior to July 1978 were generally mild. However, doses were escalated in the group of patients treated after July 1978. This was accompanied by an increase in the overall treatment time and number of fractions, with a decrease in the daily fraction size. The effect of such a change in dose-fractionation will have to be observed. However, with the biological experience (Yuhas et al.)[2] showing an increased inhibition of repair in two fraction single-cell studies, as compared to X-ray, the RBE could be increased as compared to the earlier higher daily dose schedule. Acute and intermediate reactions in this group of patients suggest that doses currently used may be within 5-10 percent of tolerance. Of the 53 patients presented here, 19 received 2700-3300 peak pion rads and 34 received more than 3300 peak pion rads. Differential effects at these two dose levels are compared below.

NORMAL TISSUE EFFECTS, ACUTE

The reactions are divided into two groups, those observed in portals re-ceiving between 2700-3300 rads, and those who received above 3300 rads of peak pions. In all sites, more numerous and more severe reactions were seen with higher doses. In the 53 patients who received 2700 peak pion rads or more, the skin was usually spared peak pion irradiation, unless the tumor was close to the skin. Occasionally, a small area of skin might be in the peak region because of the technique used in shaping the peak region with static pion beams. When dynamic treatment begins, it is expected that skin can be spared for most patients, except those in whom the skin has tumor involvement.

Evaluation of skin reactions to pions in this group is presented in Table 2.
Four patients whose skin was in the peak region, exhibited moist desquamation
of less than half the field. In all, the reactions healed rapidly. The
assessment of acute reactions to pions in 18 head and neck patients at risk is
shown in Table 3. Even the more severe reactions healed quickly. Salivary
gland suppression and loss of taste (Table 4) were noted in 14 of 18 patients
at risk, and represent the structure with the greatest degree of untoward
reactions.

Acute reactions of the rectal mucosa (Table 5) occurred in seven of the
12 patients at risk, including one with transient change in bowel habit, four
with minimal tenesmus and/or minimal injection of mucosa, one with moderate
tenesmus with mucus, and one with severe tenesmus with mucus. This latter
patient received a large boost dose, 900 peak pion rads, during the last three
days of his pion treatment. Genitourinary reactions occurred in 6 of 12
patients at risk (Table 6), and included dysuria in two, frequency in three,
and burning in one. All acute reactions of pelvic regions cleared promptly.
These reactions were mild except in two patients with frequency and dysuria.
Both of these had long histories of prostatitis, and cystoscopy revealed normal
bladder mucosa. One of the remarkable things observed with pion therapy is the
relatively moderate reaction of the rectal and bladder mucosa compared to the
amount of pelvic tumor regression. Similarly, irradiation of the abdomen for
12 pancreatic tumors was well tolerated. Two patients receiving 3000, and
3300 rads respectively, had unexplained vomiting and therefore were considered
to have radiation sickness. Two other high dose patients with liver metastases
also had nausea and vomiting. Nausea and/or vomiting was also apparent in two
of four patients treated for brain tumors. This was mild in one. In the second
patient, vomiting was relieved by aspirating the cystic center of the mass. Of
four patients receiving thoracic irradiation, two exhibited severe esophagitis,
and three acute radiation pulmonary reaction, two severe. Both cases of
esophagitis cleared fairly promptly. One of these patients had a primary
esophageal carcinoma just below the aortic arch. Radiologically the esophagus
appeared anatomically and physiologically competent, but the patient was com-
promised by an excessive intake of alcohol and died of malnutrition.
Microscopic examination of the postmortem specimen revealed no tumor.

Other acute reactions are listed in Table 7.

NORMAL TISSUE REACTIONS, LATE

Of the late reactions to pions (Table 8) the most prevalent one has been
dryness of the mouth which has persisted in 14 of 18 patients at risk. Late

TABLE 2

ACUTE REACTIONS TO PIONS - SKIN

	Peak Pion Rads	
	2700-3300	>3300
At Risk	19	34
Threshold Erythema	2	
Erythema $\geq$ 1/2 Field	8	7
Dry Desquamation < 1/2 Field	1	3
Dry Desquamation $\geq$ 1/2 Field	5	15
Moist Desquamation < 1/2 Field	1	3
TOTAL	17	28

TABLE 3

ACUTE REACTIONS TO PIONS - ORAL PHARYNGEAL

	Peak Pion Rads	
	2700-3300	>3300
At Risk	7	11
Injection	3	
Patchy Psuedo-Diphtheritic Membrane	4	8
Confluent Psuedo-Diphtheritic Membrane		3
TOTAL	7	11

TABLE 4

ACUTE REACTIONS TO PIONS - SALIVARY GLANDS

	Peak Pion Rads	
	2700-3300	>3300
At Risk	7	11
Temporary Suppression of Salivation with Dry Mouth	2	1
Partial Loss of Taste: Persistent Lack of Saliva	3	5
Complete Loss of Taste: Nonfunctioning Salivary Gland		3
TOTAL	5	9

TABLE 5

ACUTE REACTIONS TO PIONS - RECTUM

	Peak Pion Rads	
	2700-3300	>3300
At Risk	4	8
Transient Change of Bowel Habit	1	
Minimal Tenesmus and/or Reddening of Mucosa		4
Moderate Tenesmus With Mucosa		1
Severe Tenesmus With Mucus		1
TOTAL	1	6

TABLE 6

ACUTE REACTIONS TO PIONS - BLADDER

	Peak Pion Rads	
	2700-3300	>3300
At Risk	4	8
Frequency		3*
Dysuria		2
Burning		1
TOTAL	0	6

*
Cystoscopy of two cases with chronic prostatitis history showed normal bladder mucosa

TABLE 7

ACUTE REACTIONS TO PIONS - OTHERS

	Peak Pion Rads
	>3300
Epilation, Scalp	4
Nausea and Vomiting	5
Weight Loss, Excessive	3
Hemorrhage, Lingual Artery	1
Esophagitis	2
Vaginitis	1
Edema	6*

*
One case, only 3000 rads

TABLE 8

LATE EFFECTS - APPEAR OR PERSIST AFTER 6 MONTHS

	Peak Pion Rads				
	2700-3300		>3300		
	At Risk	Minimal	At Risk	Minimal	Severe
Xerostomia	7	5	11	6	3
Edema, Oral-Pharyngeal	7	1	11	2	
Dewlap	7		11	2	
Fibrosis, Subcutaneous Neck	7		9	1*	1*
Fibrosis, Lung	1		4		3
Dysuria	4		8	1	
Edema, Pelvis	4		8	1	

*
 Pions + X-ray

TABLE 9

ALIVE, STATUS WITHIN PION TREATMENT VOLUME

	Peak Pion Rads		
	2700-3300	>3300	TOTAL
At Risk	19	34	53
Local Control	5	14	19
Not Assessable	1	6	7
Disease in Treatment Volume		2	2
Regrowth in Treatment Volume	1	2	3
TOTAL	7	24	31

TABLE 10

ALIVE, STATUS OUTSIDE PION TREATMENT VOLUME

	Peak Pion Rads		
	2700-3300	>3300	TOTAL
At Risk	19	34	53
No Disease	5	19	24
Outside But Contiguous	1	1	2
Regional Metastases	1		1
Distant Metastases		4	4
TOTAL	7	24	31

edema of the mucosa has been noted in four patients and dewlap in two, while late dysuria was noted in one patient. The latter three symptoms have generally occurred at approximately 60 days after treatment and cleared by approximately 90 percent within a month or two. Serious late reaction has been fibrosis in the lung in three patients. Two of these received two palliative courses 6 and 15 months apart for a total of 4200 and 4700 peak pion rads, respectively. However, the third patient with a lung cancer in the left para-vertebral gutter received 3910 peak pion rads in 40 elapsed days, 34 fractions. She also received a severe pulmonary radiation reaction. A fourth patient was given 2700 peak pion rads in 42 elapsed days, 23 fractions and has been followed for 21 months without recurrence of his superior sulcus tumor with large mediastinal metastasis. There is no sign of fibrosis. Accordingly, the maximum dose to the coned down portion of the lung has been reduced to 3300 peak pion rads.

SURVIVAL

Thirty-one of the 53 patients who received 2700 peak pion rads or more, are alive (Tables 9-10). Of these, local control is apparent in 19, and in 7 disease is not assessable though some are probably controlled. In these seven, 3 patients had brain tumors treated five months ago, but the CT scans are not normal. Only one of the these three has intermittent symptoms. One patient with liver metastases received pion treatment to half the liver and this portion appears controlled. One patient has symptoms and signs of chronic pulmonary fibrosis which obscures the local tumor site. She has maintained her weight however, and there is no evidence of regrowth. Two patients had tongue lesions treated. There is a residual mass in each but they appear stable.

Twenty-four patients are free of disease outside of the pion treatment volume. However, two are known to have contiguous disease. One of these is the patient who purposely had only half the liver treated; the other patient had disease in regional nodes treated by conventional radiation. Four patients have distant metastases. As mentioned above, one patient with carcinoma of the esophagus died of malnutrition without any cancer cells found in the autopsy material. Another patient died one month after pion treatment of myocardial infarction, with a small residual mass in the tongue that had been planned for implant.

Twenty-two of the fifty-three patients have died (Table 11). In the peak pion volume, six had persistence, two had recurrence and one had both persistence and recurrence. Five of these local failures were in the lower dose group.

TABLE 11

PION PATIENTS DEAD

	Peak Pion Rads		
	2700-3300	>3300	TOTAL
At Risk	19	34	53
Persistence	1		1
Persistence & Recurrence		1	1
Persistence in Pion Vol. & Mets Outside	2	2	4
Recurrence in Pion Volume	2		2
Mets Outside Pion Volume	4	3	7
Complications		2	2
Infection	3		3
Intercurrent		1	1
Unknown		1	1
TOTAL	12	10	22

TABLE 12

PHASE III DOSES - PEAK PION RADS

	DAILY		TOTAL	
	MIN	MAX	MIN	MAX
Brain:				
Whole	80	100	2000	2500
Cone-Down	80	100	900	1125
Whole + Cone-Down	80	100	2900	3625
Lung:				
Mediastinum	85	106	2000	2500
Cone-Down	85	106	640	800
Mediastinum + Cone-Down	85	106	2640	3300
Larynx	85	106	2640	3300
Head & Neck (Except Larynx)	85	106	3300	4100
Abdomen	85	106	3300	4100
Pelvis	85	106	3300	4100

PLANS FOR RANDOMIZED STUDIES

Dose Schedules. A variety of time-dose schedules has been utilized due to the
schedule of operation of the accelerator at Los Alamos. With gradually length-
ening cycles, planned maintenance periods have altered. In adapting to the
schedule, both continuous and split courses have been used. Overall treatment
times varied from 32 to 59 days. With split courses the interval varied between 7 and 21 days. Except for unusual boost doses, planned daily doses have
been as high as 147 rads per day and as low as 85. Experience with acute
reactions in patients at the higher daily doses suggests the optimum daily
dose may be below a maximum of 125 rads. Most patients who received the
largest total dose (4100 pion rads) received a maximum of 106 rads daily which
yielded acceptable acute normal tissue reactions.

Based on experience to date, and the knowledge that information on
tolerance closer than $\pm$ 5 percent will require treatment of hundreds of
patients with pions, randomized trials of pion radiotherapy will begin at the
minimum dose levels defined in Table 12.

Priorities for Randomized Trials. The national advisory group for the
Los Alamos project has established priorities for randomized studies, expected
to begin in the summer of 1979. These priorities are based on (1) whether
various sites are likely to yield increased survival or local control
(both improved survival and local control are being sought in these studies),
(2) how long it is likely to take to achieve a definitive answer as to the
comparative effectiveness of pions versus x-rays, (3) whether responses are
readily assessable, and (4) expected caseload availability. The following
priorities have been assigned in order of preference for accession to the
program: (1) rectum, (2) brain, (3) head and neck, (4) pancreas, (5) prostate,
(6) bladder, and (7) larynx. Selection of patients from these sites is based
on those stages not well managed by any conventional method.

ILLUSTRATIVE CASE REPORTS

Case #39: Male, age 66, with adenocarcinoma of prostate measuring 13 cm in
diameter, Stage T3NXMO, Grade 3. Treatment began November 1977 and 3309 maximum
peak pion rads, 23 fractions, 31 days were delivered. Acute reactions to pion
therapy were dry desquamation, more than half the field; minimal tenesmus and
reddening of mucosa; and dysuria. The tumor was clinically 90 percent gone by
the end of pion therapy, and completely gone by 9 months after Day 1 of pion
therapy. Long-term effect was dysuria for approximately one year. The patient
experienced two stools per day starting approximately on Day 60 and clearing

by approximately Day 90. The patient is alive with no evidence of disease at 15 months after Day 1 of pion therapy.

Case #59: Male, age 73, with adenocarcinoma of prostate, Stage C (T2N2M1), Grade 3. The patient was treated in July–September 1978 with 4147 maximum peak pion rads, 32 fractions, 59 total elapsed days. A suspected metastatic lesion of the spine was treated with photons with a dose of 3000 rads in 9 fractions over two weeks prior to treatment with pion radiotherapy. He tolerated treatment well throughout the course, with only slight burning on urination and occasional diarrhea. He experienced mild to moderate erythema in both fields and marked shrinkage of prostatic tumor. At nine months after Day 1, the prostatic fossa was scaphoid. Neither the gland nor the previous nodularity was palpable. The suspected metastasis has shown no activity and lack of change in uptake after irradiation suggests the lesion may be other than tumor. The patient has no clinical evidence of disease.

Case #25: Male, age 64, with epidermoid carcinoma of the larynx, Stage T4N0M0, Grade 2. It was too extensive to determine point of origin but probably arose in the region of the left false cord and penetrated through the thyroid cartilage to form a contiguous mass in the left neck. The patient arrived for treatment with a tracheostomy and concomitant difficulty in breathing due to tumor pressure. Treatment started in July 1977 and he received 3000 maximum peak pion rads, 24 fractions in 44 days. Acute reactions to pion therapy were dry desquamation, more than half the field, and injection of the oral mucosa. The tracheostomy tube was removed about midway through treatment without incident. The tumor was clinically gone by the end of pion therapy. At approximately Day 60 after the start of pion therapy, the patient exhibited a mild edema of the larynx and dewlap, which cleared 90 percent within a month. Edema of the arytenoid, +1, persists. The patient is alive with no evidence of disease at 21 months after the start of pion therapy.

Case #74: Male, age 59, with squamous cell carcinoma of the left face, Stage T4N0M0. The grade was difficult to define. The patient had an excision of the tumor 12 years ago, and a second excision for recurrence two years later. The tumor again recurred at 10 years, and chemosurgery was performed. The patient was referred for pion therapy after the third recurrence two years later. At the beginning of treatment a 3.5 x 1.5 cm shallow cutaneous ulcer with a yellow necrotic membraneous base occupied the central region of the neoplasm. With supportive treatment (H_2O_2 irrigation and antibotic ointment) this ulcer nearly completely re-epithelialized _during_ therapy even though it was within the region of the peak pion maximum dose. X-ray examination revealed involvement of the zygoma. He underwent pion radiotherapy in November-December 1978, with 3870 maximum peak pion rads, 39 fractions, 52 elapsed days. He exhibited a dry desquamation of the skin, more than half the field; patchy pseudo-diphtheritic membrane of the oral mucosa, more than half the field; and suppression of saliva with dry mouth. Before treatment, edema was present around the left eye due to the tumor, but was exacerbated during treatment. At the end of treatment, it was estimated that the tumor was 90 percent smaller, with the ulcer reduced to less than 1 cm. One month after treatment the ulcer was gone and there was no evidence of disease. The cosmetic effect was remarkably good. The patient is alive and free of disease at four months after the start of pion therapy.

Case #61: Female, age 22, with symptoms of a rapidly growing malignant tumor of the frontal lobe (Astrocytoma Grade III, histologic grade 3). The patient was sent for pion therapy after minimal surgical decompression. She was treated with 4109 maximum peak pion rads, 37 fractions, 62 days, in July-September 1978. Within days, she experienced symptomatic improvement and continued to improve during and after pion therapy. Acute reactions included complete epilation of the scalp, dry desquamation of the skin, more than half the field, and nausea and vomiting toward the end of treatment. She also lost about 10 pounds due in part to an acute viral respiratory illness. CT scan midway through treatment showed partial tumor regression (approximately 25 percent), and she continued to do well until six months after the start of pion therapy, when her symptoms returned. CT scan at that time indicated a possible recurrence in the center of the tumor volume. On 2/1/79 she received 160 mg of CCNU, and 120 mg on 4/5/79. The reduced dose was given because of a drop in platelets. However, she has experienced minimal side effects. She is working, but does have intermittent episodes of rightsided weakness relieved by short courses of Decadron. The patient is alive nine months after the start of pion radiotherapy.

REFERENCES

1. Hogstrom, K.R.; Smith, A.R.; Kelsey, C.A.; Simon, S.L.; Somers, J.W.; Lane, R.G.; Rosen, I.I.; von Essen, C.F.; Kligerman, M.M.; Berardo, P.A.; and Zink, S.M.: Static pion beam treatment planning of deep seated tumors using computerized tomography scans at LAMPF. International Journal of Radiation Oncology, Biology, and Physics, in press.

2. Yuhas, J.; Li, A., and Kligerman, M.: Present status of the proposed use of negative pi mesons in radiotherapy. In: Advances in Radiation Biology, Vol. 8, in press. Academic Press, New York. Editor, John Lett.

© 1979, Elsevier/North-Holland Biomedical Press
Treatment of Radioresistant Cancers
M. Abe, K. Sakamoto and T.L. Phillips eds.

RADIOBIOLOGICAL BASIS FOR HEAVY-ION THERAPY

C. A. TOBIAS, E. A. ALPEN, E. A. BLAKELY, J. R. CASTRO, A. CHATTERJEE,

G.T.Y. CHEN, S. B. CURTIS, J. HOWARD, J. T. LYMAN, AND F.Q.H. NGO

Division of Biology and Medicine, Lawrence Berkeley Laboratory, University
of California, Berkeley, California 94720, U.S.A.

INTRODUCTION

A systematic investigation of the potential therapeutic usefulness of
accelerated nuclei is in progress at the Lawrence Berkeley Laboratory.
Particles of atomic numbers ranging from 6 to 26 and kinetic energies up
to 1 GeV/amu are available in the biomedical facility. These particles
combine physical and radiobiological advantages in a unique manner. Some
of the particles can have depth dose distributions comparable to, or in some
instances better than, protons, helium ions, pi mesons, or fast neutron dose
distributions. At the same time the heavier particles markedly reduce the
radiobiological oxygen effect to a degree comparable to the best levels
achievable with neutrons.

In 1946 Robert Wilson first suggested that beams of atomic nuclei[1] may
have therapeutic usefulness. The initial biological experiments with deuterons,
and the first human therapeutic use with protons were performed at Berkeley
by Tobias, Lawrence et al.[2,3] The HILAC accelerator later became a source
of heavy particles for cell biology.[4] Over a period of twenty years helium
ions at Berkeley and protons at Harvard were used with considerable success
for pituitary radiation therapy of acromegaly and of Cushing's disease.[5]
Tobias and Todd suggested the therapeutic use of heavier ions in 1967[6], and
the rationale was then worked out in some detail.[7,8]

In 1971 it was demonstrated at the Princeton synchrotron[9] and at the Berkeley
Bevatron[10] that large synchrotrons designed for proton acceleration are also
suitable for accelerating nitrogen and other heavy nuclei. The Berkeley
Bevalac, a new accelerator complex consisting of the Bevatron with the HILAC
as an injector, was completed in 1975.[11] All the work described here was

done with the Bevalac. With joint support by the U. S. Department of Energy and the National Cancer Institute, systematic biomedical research and therapy are now being performed with about 50% of the research done by members of our laboratory and 50% by visiting scientists from many laboratories around the world. I am pleased to report that we already have one Japanese scientist, Dr. N. Takata of the Electrotechnical Laboratory, working on secondary electron production by heavy particles at the Bevalac. In addition, we hope we will soon have a joint U.S.-Japan program to encourage a larger degree of cooperative research in investigating the effects of accelerated ions.

PHYSICAL ADVANTAGES OF HEAVY-ION BEAMS FOR THERAPY

The physical advantages of heavy-ion beams for therapy can be divided into three fields:

1. It is possible to maximize the biologically effective dose in the tumor while maintaining low biologically effective dose levels at the entrance and exit ports. This affords considerable protection to radiosensitive normal tissues lying inside the exposure field, but outside the tumor target region.

2. The new technique of heavy-ion radiography allows visualization of soft tissue tumors in many instances with greater sensitivity than can be achieved with other currently available techniques. We anticipate that heavy-ion radiography will become an important adjunct to tumor localization and therapy planning.

3. In the future radioactive beams will be used in conjunction with positron cameras to directly observe the region where therapy beam particles stop in human tissue. Thus, the use of radioactive beams will allow verification of radiation treatment plans.

THE PHYSICS OF THERAPY BEAMS

The Bevalac usually produces monoenergetic nearly parallel particle beams. The particles are delivered in 15 pulses per minute; each pulse is a few tenths of a second long. The beam energy is determined by the exact timing of the beam spill during the acceleration cycle, and the beams are further shaped and directed by sets of quadrupole and deflecting magnets. In cross section the particles form a two-dimensional gaussian distribution; the mean radius can be varied from about 0.5 cm to about 20 cm. The dose rate is adequate. A tumor of 1 liter volume $(10 \text{ cm})^3$ can be treated with carbon, neon, or argon particles at a dose rate of 100 rad/min or higher.

Figure 1 shows the Bragg ionization curve of a monoenergetic neon beam in water. The ionization peak occurs just before the particles are stopping. The overall ionization curve can be analyzed into two parts; the ionization due to the primary beam particles and the ionization due to fragments formed by nuclear collisions along the pathway of the beam.

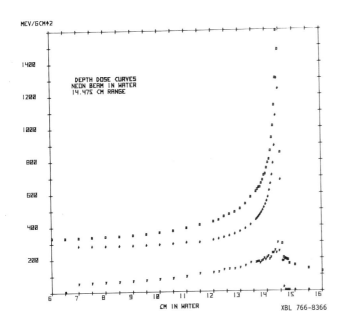

MEV/GCM*2

DEPTH DOSE CURVES
NEON BEAM IN WATER
14.475 CM RANGE

CM IN WATER   XBL 766-8366

Fig. 1. Bragg ionization curve of a neon beam in water: (□) total ionization, (+) primary beam; (y) fragments.

The linear energy transfer (LET) of the particles changes with depth and is generally highest very near the stopping point of each particle. Thus, the biological effect at each depth is due to a dose and LET distribution. This is especially true for the ridge filtered beams which are used in therapy. Part of the radiological physics effort is directed to finding optimal designs for filters. If we delivered uniform dose everywhere in the tumor, the biological effect would still vary from one location to the next due to the fact that the LET distribution is different in each location. Our goals are: (a) to produce isoeffect in the tumor, and (b) to reduce as much as possible the dose to normal tissues lying in the entrance or exit fields. Once these goals are achieved, we wish to design particle distributions that also minimize uniformly the radiobiological oxygen effect in the tumor target region.

At the present time mixed beam radiation is achieved by passing the mono-energetic therapy beams through a spiral ridge filter. The filters are usually made of brass, and a series of ridges are precisely machined in a spiral fashion. The filter rapidly rotates in a plane perpendicular to the axis of the beam. The shape of the filter determines the particle mix in the therapy beam. This type of filter was earlier used for protons at Uppsala.[12] Figure 2 shows a variety of dose and LET distributions when the shape of the filter is an exponentially decreasing function of the distance between ridges. By changing the slope of the exponent one obtains a variety of depth-dose shapes (see the upper panel of Figure 2). At the same time, the mean LET distribution becomes increasingly (but not completely) uniform (see the lower panel of Figure 2).

On the basis of mammalian cell survival data, Lyman designed a set of ridge filters which are currently used in therapy.[13] In Figure 3, dose and calculated effect distributions are shown for a set of isosurvival filters. In order to obtain isoeffect, the physical dose distribution has a character-istic "ramp" feature, shown in the central panel of Figure 3. To optimize effective dose distributions for each particle and for each energy, a different set of filters has been designed for a range of tumor dimensions.

It is not possible to obtain isosurvival for both aerobic and hypoxic cells simultaneously with a single port exposure of a heavy-ion beam. The simplest way to achieve such conditions is by crossfiring beams--two parallel opposed port ridge filtered particle beams with appropriate overlap in the tumor regions. Another more complicated alternative is the multiport or rotational approach.

HEAVY-ION RADIOGRAPHY

Since this method has been described elsewhere[14,15] we wish to mention it only briefly here. Figure 4 shows isoelectron density contours obtained by computer reconstruction of carbon-ion radiographs of a patient who received helium-ion treatments concurrently for pancreatic carcinoma. The contour

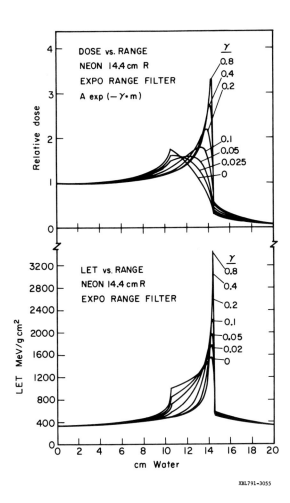

Fig. 2. Dose and mean LET variation in depth for a variety of range filters. The thickness of these filters varies as an exponential function. Top: dose distributions for a 4-cm range filter at various values of gamma. Bottom: LET distributions for various gamma values.

164

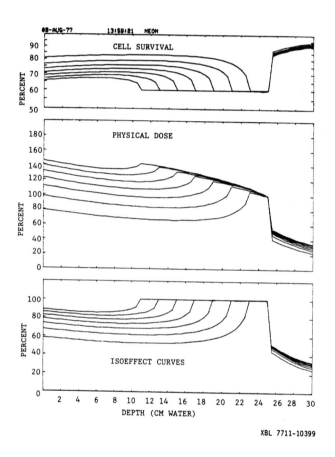

Fig. 3. <u>Top</u>: calculated cell survival for "typical" mammalian cells. <u>Center</u>: depth-dose distributions for filters used in therapy and research (neon beam). <u>Bottom</u>: isoeffect curves.

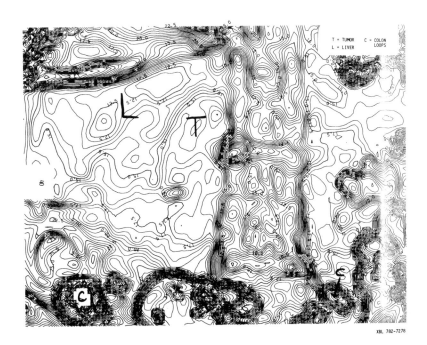

Fig. 4. Isoelectron density plot obtained by carbon radiography as described
in the text. (L) liver; (T) tumor; (C) colon loops.

plot shows the spinal column, lung, loops of the colon (C), the liver (L),
and   the region of the tumor (T). This radiograph was taken by W. Holley
and J. Fabrikant. The exact stopping power value of the contours is of
definite interest since these show the thickness of the structures in appropriate electronic stopping power units. We are currently engaged in cross
calibrating the stopping power measured in carbon-ion radiographs with
stopping power calculations from x-ray computerized tomography. It is
necessary to do this for accurate placement of the heavy ion therapy beams.

RADIOACTIVE BEAMS

   Radioactive beams are obtained when the nonradioactive primary beam collides
with absorber nuclei.[16,17] We have observed $^{11}_{6}C$ in carbon beams, $^{15}_{8}O$ in
$^{16}_{8}O$ beams, and $^{19}_{10}Ne$ in $^{20}_{10}Ne$ beams. J. Alonso et al.[18] were able to separate

the radioactive beam from the parent beam, due to the fact that these have different charge to mass ratios. Figure 5 shows the Bragg ionization curve of a $^{19}_{10}$Ne beam separated from $^{20}_{10}$Ne. This beam is relatively free of $^{20}_{10}$Ne; however, it does have some $^{17}_{9}$F and $^{15}_{8}$O contamination.

A special positron camera has been constructed by J. Llacer and A. Chatterjee. At the expense of about a 5 rad dose, the stopping point of a monoenergetic beam has been determined to 0.1 cm accuracy by the camera in the time span of a few seconds.

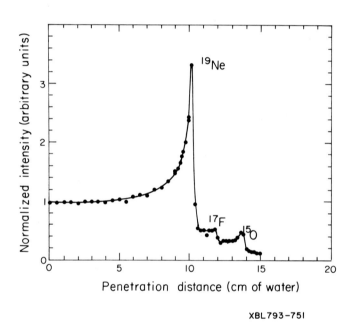

XBL793-751

Fig. 5. Bragg ionization curve of a ^{19}Ne beam magnetically separated from the parent ^{20}Ne beam.

Figure 6 is an artist's drawing of the manner in which the radioactive beams might be deployed in the future to monitor depth penetration of the beam during therapy planning procedures, and perhaps even during actual therapy. It is particularly easy to monitor small beams stopping in the head and neck region. We anticipate that in the future, the carbon-ion beam might be used for Bragg peak therapy of the pituitary gland.

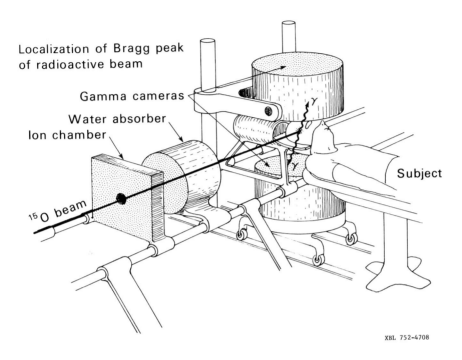

Localization of Bragg peak
of radioactive beam

Gamma cameras

Water absorber

Ion chamber

Subject

^{15}O beam

XBL 752-4708

Fig. 6. Schematic drawing for possible future use of radioactive beams. A monoenergetic ^{15}O beam is used to deliver a therapeutic dose to the pituitary gland. A positron camera continually monitors the depth penetration of the beam.

THERAPY PLANNING

The properties of heavy-ion beams make expert therapy planning mandatory. Chen and Lyman are developing a computerized treatment planning method.[19] Quantitative stopping power data, calculated from x-ray tomograms, are used for calculating isodose curves. The heavy-ion beam properties are also in the computer memory. Figure 7 (A,B) shows two of the steps in the procedure. Figure 7A is a CAT scan of a patient with pancreatic carcinoma. Figure 7B shows the same scan transferred to the therapy planning computer. A three port approach is used. The numbers shown on Figure 7B are dose levels in CoRE units (cobalt rad equivalent). The kidneys and spinal cord are protected. The plan shown here was for helium ions.

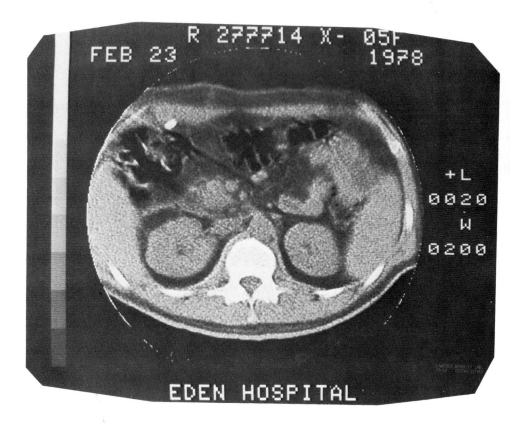

Fig. 7A. A computerized x-ray tomogram of the midsection of a patient with pancreatic carcinoma.

Initial human application

Until May 1979, about 150 cancer patients were treated with helium ions and 18 patients had received carbon, neon, or argon beam therapy. Dosimetry was based on the considerations given above and on pretherapeutic studies using cells in culture and tissue radiobiology experience. Initial tasks include verification of the RBE factors, establishing the degree of human tissue tolerance to heavy charged particle beams, and comparison of the RBE factors gained in pretherapeutic studies to those obtainable for humans. Initial impressions are that the dosimetry and biological studies were adequate. Because of the good dose distribution curves, normal tissues surrounding the tumors are spared, and patients tolerate heavy-ion radiation well.

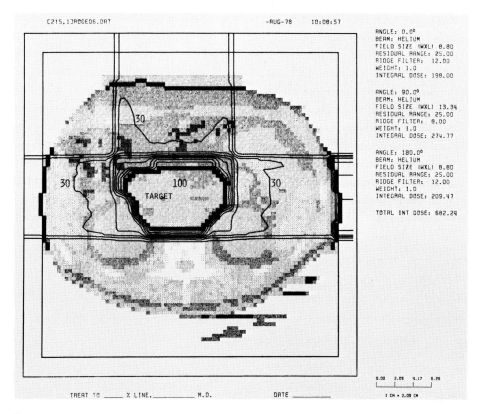

Fig. 7B. The CAT scan transferred to the therapy planning computer. A three port approach is used. Isodose curves are shown.

Under the auspices of the Radiation Therapy Oncology Group (RTOG) and the Northern California Oncology Group (NCOG), we are planning controlled therapy studies. Several classes of tumors are being considered for inclusion in the randomized studies. Initial experience is available with pancreatic carcinoma, brain tumors, tumors of the head and neck, and gastric tumors. J. Castro is chairman of the Bay Area Heavy Ion Association (BAHIA). This is a group of physicians and scientists who are participants in these therapy oriented studies.

RADIOBIOLOGICAL CONSIDERATIONS

One reason there is much interest in the therapeutic application of heavy ions is the demonstrated fact that at low particle velocities and at very high LET the radiobiological oxygen effect becomes very small.[20,21] As radiobiological investigations have progressed, we have become aware of additional factors that may contribute to the therapeutic efficacy of these particles. Some of these are listed in Figure 8. We shall briefly discuss several of these factors.

CELLULAR RADIOBIOLOGICAL RESULTS
OF
POTENTIAL THERAPEUTIC SIGNIFICANCE

1. RBE ↑

2. OER ↓

3. Aneuploid cell line sensitivity ↑

4. Age response ↓

5. Profound G_2 block

6. H.I. produce lethal and
   nonlethal lesions

7. Cell contact protection ↓

8. Fractionation and mixed modality
   gain factors

XBL791-3035

Fig. 8. A list of radiobiological factors of potential significance in heavy-ion therapy.

Increased biological effectiveness at low velocities

Most mammalian cell curvival curves when exposed to low LET radiation are of the multihit type; in other words, survival curves have "shoulders." The cells of radioresistant tissues and tumors usually have large shoulders in their survival curves. In heavy-ion survival curves, an initial exponential component helps to reduce the shoulder. For very high LET, that is for particles of high atomic number and low velocity, mammalian survival curves are essentially exponential. Since the "shoulders" on survival curves are

often associated with enzymatic repair of radiolesions, it is generally
believed that the lesions produced by heavy ions are less repairable than
those produced by x rays. We have discussed these phenomena in the repair-
misrepair model.[22]

E. Blakely et al.[23] studied survival of human kidney cells in monolayer
culture when these were exposed to a variety of heavy ion beams. The summary
of her results are shown in Figure 9, where the relative biological effectiveness (RBE) is shown as a function of residual range for carbon, neon, and
argon ions. Where the RBE is high, the survival curves are generally more
exponential; where the RBE is low, they show shoulders. The RBE for each
of the particles is higher near the Bragg peak than at the plateau of the
ionization curves. In therapy use, this type of RBE dependence on particle
range helps to increase the biological effect at the extended Bragg peak
in tumors, and to decrease the effects at the plateau where the beams enter
the body.

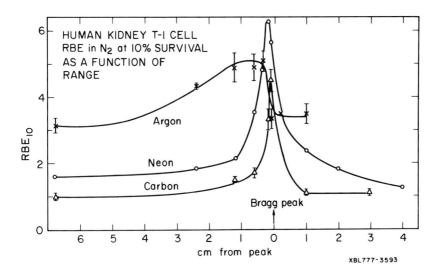

XBL777-3593

Fig. 9. Relative biological effectiveness as a function of residual range for
human T-1 kidney cells. The values given are for 10% survival levels. The
effects of fragments are included.

The increased biological effectiveness of heavy ions has been demonstrated for many different systems and for various end points.[24-31]

Using a rodent tumor system in vivo, a rat rhabdomyosarcoma, Curtis et al.[32] measured growth delay in the plateau and extended Bragg peak for various beams. These results are shown in Figure 10. The relative biological effectiveness for growth delay is comparable to that observed for inhibition of cell division.

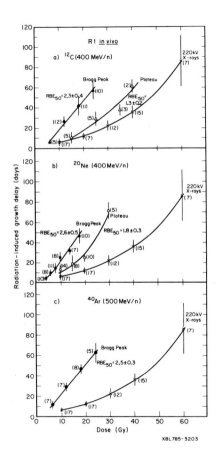

Fig. 10. Heavy-ion radiation induced growth delay in rat rhabdomyosarcoma tumors. X-ray effects, and particle beam plateau and extended peak are shown separately.

Oxygen enhancement ratio (OER)

Localized radioresistant tumors with poor circulation have many anoxic cells and sometimes even necrotic centers are present. Such tumors are candidates for heavy-ion particle therapy. Blakely[23] has measured the oxygen enhancement ratio for the various particles and a summary of her data are shown in Figure 11. Each of the heavy particles have reduced OER near the Bragg peak. For argon beams, the oxygen effect ratio is materially reduced for several cm of residual range. Experiments with extended Bragg peaks, using human kidney cells[33], have allowed plotting of depth survival curves in Figure 12 using appropriate ridge filters and the crossfire technique. Dose levels have been chosen in such a manner that in the extended Bragg peak 10% of aereated cells would survive after a single dose. The major difference in the three sets of curves is that hypoxic cell survival is much lower with argon than with other beams. Note that the entrance dose to produce the same depth effect is progressively less for heavier particles.

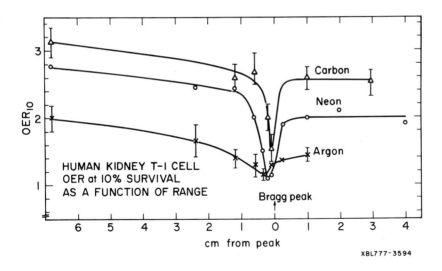

XBL777-3594

Fig. 11. Oxygen enhancement ratio (OER) as a function of residual range. The OER for argon ions is consistently the lowest.

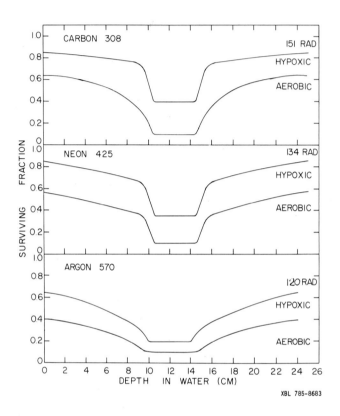

Fig. 12. Human kidney cell depth survival curves following crossfire of carbon, neon, and argon beams for hypoxic and aerated cells. The oxygen effect in the "tumor" is smallest for argon.

In an independent set of experiments by Curtis et al.[34] the RBE and OER were measured in 10 cm extended Bragg peaks of carbon, neon, and argon beams for rhabdomyosarcoma cells in suspension. For this system, the argon particles also produce much lower OER values than neon, carbon, or x rays. For the entire extended peak the argon OER was between 1.2 and 1.45 (see Figure 13). It appears that of the particles tested, argon is most effective in lowering the oxygen effect. We wish to make further experiments with silicon or perhaps phosphorus beams; these fragment less than argon but should still have a low OER.

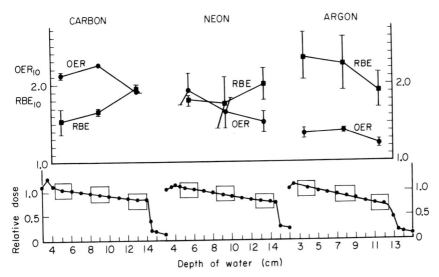

RHABDOMYOSARCOMA CELLS IN SUSPENSION

XBL795-3436

Fig. 13.   RBE and OER values for rat rhabdomyosarcoma cells in vitro.   A 10-cm extended Bragg peak was used.   The OER is lowest for argon.

Chapman found that electron affinic radiosensitizers have about the same effectiveness when used with heavy ions as they do with x rays.[31,35]   Their use lowers the OER, thus, combined therapeutic use of heavy ions and radiosensitizers is a distinct future possibility.

Aneuploid cell line sensitivity

It is known that the general magnitude of cell sensitivity to ionizing radiations is a function of DNA content.   Cells with greater amounts of DNA appear to be more sensitive.   We know, however, that there are many factors that modify sensitivity including genetic and physiological factors.   We have compared the radiation sensitivity of two cell lines: hamster V79 cells and human kidney T-1 cells.   The hamster strain is near diploid, and has 22 pairs of chromosomes.   The kidney cells are aneuploid; they have between

60 and 80 chromosome pairs and more DNA than the hamster cells. Figure 14
shows the dependence of RBE on LET when accelerated argon ions are used.
At the 50% survival level the human kidney cells are much more sensitive
to particles above 140 keV/ m than hamster cells. The peak RBE is reached
for hamster cells at a lower LET than for the kidney cells. At the 10%
survival level these differences vanish. The effect is greatest for the
low dose exponential part of the survival curves. More work is obviously
necessary in order to compare the radiosensitivity of normal human diploid
cells and human tumor cell lines. Many tumors are known to have hyperploid
and aneuploid cells, therefore, it appears reasonable to assume that these
cells are more sensitive at low dose to very high-LET radiation than normal
cells are.

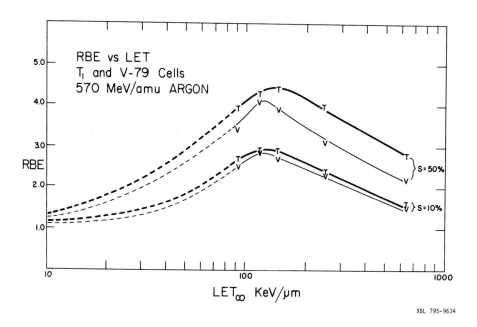

XBL 795-9634

Fig. 14. LET dependence of the relative biological effectiveness for human
kidney cells and hamster V79 cells, measured with argon beams. The RBE for
V79 cells has a peak at lower LET than for human kidney cells. At 50% survival
the effect is marked; at 10% survival the effect is not significant.

E. Blakely plotted the RBE for mammalian cells in vitro as function of
LET and compared the results for mammalian cell systems studied in vivo by
various investigators. These results are shown in Figure 15. There is a
great deal of scatter in the data, nevertheless, it is apparent that the
tissues studied in vivo have their maximum RBE at a considerably lower LET
(~100 keV/μm) than cells in culture (~150 keV/μm). The cell isolates consisted of human kidney cells, rat cells, mouse tumor cells, and hamster cells.
The techniques used for in vivo observations of tissue sensitivity are very
different from those used for tissue culture. Nevertheless, we believe that
more studies are needed to elucidate the differences in sensitivities of
normal tissues and tumor cells to heavy ions.

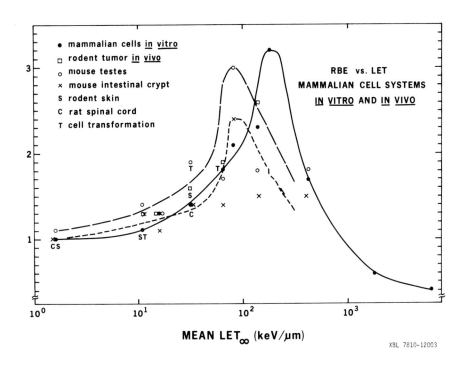

XBL 7810-12003

Fig. 15. RBE vs LET studied by heavy ions. The peak of the RBE curve for
tissues in vivo is shifted to the left when compared to mammalian cells studied
in vitro. (——) mammalian cells in culture; (— — —) and (- - -) mammalian
tissues in vivo.

Cell age response to heavy ions

It is well known that cells are most radioresistant to x rays when they are in late S phase, whereas they are most sensitive in G2, M, and the G1S boundary stages. When heavy ions are used the differences in sensitivity between the various physiological states are greatly diminished.

For kidney cells at 2% survival level, cell cycle survival variations are less than 2.5 times for argon beams, whereas they are about tenfold for x rays. Hall[29] and Raju[36] both found less than twofold variation for argon beams when V79 and Chinese hamster ovary cells were used.

When a population of exponentially growing tumor cells is compared to normal differentiated tissues, the S phase of the tumor cells might be most resistant to x rays. In protracted radiation schedules the tumor cells would be better protected because at any given time there would be some cells in S phase. The importance to radiotherapy has been discussed by Withers.[37]

Accumulation of cells in G2 stage

C. Lücke-Hühle[38] measured the DNA content of V79 hamster cells to study cell progression following exposure to heavy ions. At about 8 hours post-irradiation she found that many cells were blocked in the radiosensitive G2 stage. The effect for heavy ions is greater than for x rays, and the RBE for G2 block is higher than for survival. Mammalian cells are more sensitive to a second dose of irradiation during the G2 stage, and this finding might give important clues for the strategy of dose fractionation with heavy ions.

Sublethal lesions produced by heavy ions

We have shown above that the survival response to heavy ions usually has an initial exponential portion. This part of survival curves are usually interpreted by assuming that a single charged particle, passing through the cell nucleus causes inhibition of reproductive integrity. F. Ngo has recently shown that sublethal lesions are produced by heavy ions in cells that are not killed by a single hit.[39] An initial dose of neon ions, for example, sensitizes the cells to a subsequent dose of x rays.[40] The sublethal lesions produced by heavy ions can be repaired, although this repair appears to be slower than the repair of x ray induced radiolesions. Thus, mixed modalities can be in some instances nearly as effective as complete dose schedules of heavy ions.

Potentiation by heavy ions

When split doses of heavy ions are given with a time interval between them, one may observe that the first dose potentiates the effects of the second. Ngo observed this effect with V79 cells irradiated with very high LET particles, such as neon, at the Bragg peak.[41] The existence of this effect is an indication that in protracted therapeutic dose schedules the effectiveness of heavy particles might be greater than can be obtained from single acute exposures.

Cell contact protection

The proximity of cells in tissues sometimes seems to evoke repair mechanisms that are not usually seen with cell isolates in vitro.[42] Thus, cells of an intact tissue can be more resistant to radiation than individual cells. When cells are grown in spheroid cultures, some strains show increased radio-resistance as evidenced by a greater shoulder on their survival curve. We do not know at this time whether this effect is due to the nutritional state of the cell, the accumulation of waste products, the accumulation of cells in G1 stage, or to genuine cell-to-cell communication. Some cell strains exhibit this protection and others do not, but we know that genetic factors are involved. Lücke-Hühle, and Rodriquez and Alpen, found marked cell contact protection to x rays; heavy ions, however, diminished and eliminated this effect. [43,44]

SUMMARY

During the last four years, many physical and radiobiological data have been obtained with accelerated heavy ions at the Berkeley Bevalac. It was demonstrated that carbon, neon, and argon ions combine the physical advantages of good depth-dose distribution with the biological advantages of low OER and high RBE in the tumor region. Argon beams have the lowest OER while carbon gives the best depth-dose advantages. Other radiobiological factors that may contribute to the therapeutic efficacy of heavy-ion beams are: reduced cell sensitivity variation during the cell division cycle and the blockage of cell progression in the radiosensitive G2 phase. Aneuploid cells appear to be more sensitive to heavy ions than euploid cells. Heavy ions produce sublethal lesions for x rays. Repair between split doses of heavy-ions is reduced, and sometimes one finds enhancement of radiobiological effects when very high LET particles are used.

Heavy-ion radiography and the use of radioactive beams offer diagnostic advantages for tumor localization and therapy planning. A controlled series of studies on heavy-ion therapy of certain tumor classes is in its beginning stage.

The Bevalac is a national facility. Qualified scientists are invited to propose experiments meaningful to the cancer problem.

ACKNOWLEDGEMENTS

These studies were supported by the National Cancer Institute (USA), and the Office of Health and Environmental Research of the U. S. Department of Energy under contract No. W-7405-ENG-48.

REFERENCES

1. Wilson, R. R. (1946). Radiological use of fast protons. Radiology, 47, 487-491.

2. Tobias, C. A., Anger, H. O., and Lawrence, J. H. (1952) Radiological use of high energy deuterons and alpha particles. Am. J. Roentgenol. Rad. Ther. Nucl. Med., 67, 1-27.

3. Tobias, C. A., Lawrence, J. H., Born, J. L., McCombs, R. K., Roberts, J. E., Anger, H. O., Low-Beer, B.V.A., and Higgins, C. B. (1958) Pituitary irradiation with high-energy proton beams: A preliminary report. Cancer Res., 18, 121-134.

4. Sayeg, J. A., Birge, A. C., Beam, C. A., and Tobias, C. A. (1959) The effects of accelerated carbon nuclei and other radiations on the survival of haploid yeast. II. Biological experiments. Radiat. Res., 10, 449-461.

5. Tobias, C. A. (1979) Pituitary radiation: radiation physics and biology. In Proceedings, International Symposium on the Recent Advances in the Diagnosis and Treatment of Pituitary Tumors,

6. Tobias, C. A. and Todd P. W. (1967) Heavy charged particles in cancer therapy. In Radiobiology and Radiotherapy. U. S. National Cancer Monograph 24. National Cancer Institute, Bethesda, MD.

7. Tobias, C. A., Lyman, J. T., and Lawrence, J. H. (1971) Some considerations of physical and biological factors in radiotherapy with high-LET radiations including heavy particles, pi mesons, and fast neutrons. In Progress in Atomic Medicine: Recent Advances in Nuclear Medicine, 3, 167-218. Grune and Stratton, New York.

8. Tobias, C. A. (1973) Pretherapeutic investigations with accelerated heavy ions. Radiology, 108, 145-158.

9. White, M. G., Isaila, M., and Prelec, K. (1971) Acceleration of nitrogen ions to 7.4 GeV in the Princeton particle accelerator. Science, 174, 1121-1123.

10. Grunder, H. A., Hartsough, W. D., and Lofgren, E. D. (1971) Acceleration of heavy ions at the Bevatron. Science, 174, 1128-1129.

11. Ghiorso, A., Grunder, H., Hartsough, W., Lambertson, G., Lofgren, E., Lou, K., Main, R., Mobley, R., Morgado, R., Salsig, W., and Selph, F. (1973) The Bevalac: An economical facility for very high energetic heavy particle research. IEEE Trans. Nucl. Sci. NS-20, 155.

12. Karlsson, B. G. (1964) Methoden zur Berechnung und Erzielurg liniger fuer die Tiefentherapie mit hochenergetischen Proteonen guenstiger Dosiverteilungen. Strahlentherapie, 124, 481-492.

13. Lyman, J. T. and Howard, J. (1977) Dosimetry and instrumentation for helium and heavy ions. Int. J. Radiat. Oncol. Biol. Phys., 3, 81-85.

14. Tobias, C. A., Benton, E. V., and Capp, M. P. (1978) Heavy-ion radiography. In Recent Advances in Nuclear Medicine, 5, 71-102. Grune and Stratton, New York.

15. Sommer, F. G., Capp, M. P., Tobias, C. A., Benton, E. V., Woodruff, K. H., Henke, R. P., Holley, W. R., and Genant, H. K. (1978) Heavy-ion radiography Density Resolution and specimen radiography. Invest. Radiol., 13, 163-170.

16. Tobias, C. A., Chatterjee, A., and Smith, A. R. (1971) Radioactive fragmentation of N-7+ ion beam observed in a beryllium target. Phys. Lett., 73A, 119.

17. Chatterjee, A. and Tobias, C. A. (1977) Radioactive beams. In Biological and Medical Research with Accelerated Heavy Ions 1974-1977. Lawrence Berkeley Laboratory Report LBL-5610, pp. 59-75.

18. Alonso, J. R., Chatterjee, A., and Tobias, C. A. (1979) High purity radioactive beams at the Bevalac. IEEE Trans. Nucl. Sci., 26, 3003.

19. Chen, G.T.Y., Castro, J. R., Lyman J. T., Quivey, J. M., Singh, R. P., and Pitluck. S. (1978) Computerized treatment planning with heavy ions. Int. J. Radiat. Oncol. Biol. Phys., 4, 203.

20. Todd, P. W. (1964) Reversible and irreversible effects of ionizing radiations on the reproductive integrity of mammalian cells cultured in vitro. Ph.D. Thesis, University of California, Berkeley.

21. Barendsen, G. W. (1968) Responses of cultured cells, tumors, and normal tissues to radiations of different linear energy transfer. In Current Topics in Radiation Research, M. Ebert and A. Howard, eds., vol. IV, pp. 293-356. North Holland Publishing Co., Amsterdam.

22. Tobias, C. A., Blakely, E. A., Ngo, F.Q.H., and Yang, T.C.H. (1979) The repair-misrepair model of cell survival. Proceedings, 32nd Annual Symposium on Fundamental Cancer Research, 26 February to 1 March 1979, Houston, Texas. In press.

23. Blakely, E. A., Tobias, C. A., Yang, T.C.H., Smith, K. C., and Lyman, J. T. (1979) Inactivation of human kidney cells by high-energy mono-energetic heavy-ion beams. Radiat. Res., in press.

24. Raju, M. R., Amols, H. I., Bain, E., Carpenter, S. G., Cox, R. A., and Robertson, J. B. (1978) A heavy particle comparative study. Part III. OER and RBE. Br. J. Radiol., 51, 712-719.

25. Raju, M. R., and Carpenter, S. G. (1978) A heavy particle comparative study. Part IV. Acute and late reactions. Br. J. Radiol., 51, 720-727.

182

26. Leith, J. T., Arcellana, V., Lyman, J. T., and Wheeler, K. T. (1975)
    Response of a rat brain tumour to irradiation with accelerated neon
    ions. Int. J. Radiat. Biol., 28, 91-97.

27. Leith, J. T., Woodruff, K. H., Lewinsky, B. S., Lyman, J. T., and Tobias,
    C. A. (1975) Tolerance of the spinal cord of rats to irradiation with
    neon ions. Int. J. Radiat. Biol., 28, 393-398.

28. Leith, J. T., Woodruff, K. H., and Lyman, J. T. (1976) Early effects
    of single doses of 375 MeV/nucleon 20-neon ions on the skin of mice
    and hamsters. Radiat. Res., 65, 440-450.

29. Hall, E. J., Bird, R. P., Rossi, H. H., Coffey, R., Varga, J., and Lam,
    Y. M. (1977) Biophysical studies with high energy arton ions. 2.
    Determiniation of the relative biological effectiveness, the oxygen
    enhancement ratio, and the cell cycle response. Radiat. Res., 70, 469-
    479.

30. Chapman, J. D., Blakely, E. A., Smith, K. C., and Urtasun, R. C. (1977)
    Radiobiological characterization of the inactivating events produced
    in mammalian cells by helium and heavy ions. Int. J. Radiat. Oncol.
    Biol. Phys., 3, 97-102.

31. Fu, K. and Phillips, T. (1976) The relative biological effectiveness
    and oxygen enhancement ratio of neon ions for the EMT6 tumor. Radiology,
    120, 439-441.

32. Curtis, S. B., Tenforde, T. S., Parks, D., Schilling, W. A., and Lyman,
    J. T. (1978) Response of a rat rhabdomyosarcoma to neon and helium
    ion irradiation. Radiat. Res., 74, 274-288.

33. Blakely, E. A., Tobias, C. A., Ngo, F.Q.H., Yang, T.C.H., Smith, K.
    C., Chang, P. Y., and Yezzi, M. J. (1978) Comparison of helium and
    heavy-ion beams for therapy based on cellular radiobiological data.
    Int. J. Radiat. Oncol. Biol. Phys., 4, 93.

34. Schilling, W. A., Curtis, S. B., Tenforde, T. S., Crabtree, K. E.,
    Lyman, J. T., and Howard. J. (1977) Comparison of the radiation response
    of rat tumor cells exposed at various positions in the extended Bragg
    peak of heavy-ion beams. Radiat. Res., 70, 642.

35. Chapman, J. D., Urtasun, R. C., Blakely, E. A., Smith, K. C., and Tobias,
    C. A. (1978) Hypoxic cell sensitizers and heavy charged particle radia-
    tions. Br. J. Cancer, 37, 184-188.

36. Raju, M. R., Bain, E., Carpenter, S., and Walters, R. A. (1979) Effects
    of argon ions on synchronized cells. Proceedings, Sixth International
    Congress of Radiation Research, May 1979, Tokyo, Japan.

37. Withers, H. R. (1973) Biological basis for high LET radiotherapy.
    Radiology,108, 131-137.

38. Lücke-Hühle, C., Blakely, E. A., Chang, P. Y., and Tobias, C. A. (1979)
    Drastic G2 arrest in mammalian cells after irradiation with heavy-ion
    beams. Radiat. Res., in press.

39. Ngo, F.A.H., Blakely, E. A., and Tobias, C. A. (1978) Does an exponential
    survival curve of irradiation mammalian cells imply no repair? Radiat.
    Res., 74, 588.

40. Ngo, F.Q.H., Blakely, E. A., and Tobias, C. A. Low and high-LET radiations do not act independently. I. Evidence of repairable damage in asynchronous V79 hamster cells after high-energy neon charged particles. Submitted to Radiat. Res.

41. Ngo, F.Q.H., Blakely, E. A., Tobias, C. A., Chang, P. Y., and Smith, K. C. (1978) Fractionation gain factor from therapetic heavy-ion beams. Int. J. Radiat. Oncol. Biol. Phys., 4, 92.

42. Sutherland, R. M. and Durand, R. E. (1976) Radiation response of multicell spheroids: An in vitro tumor model. Curr. Topics Radiat. Res. Q., 11, 87-139.

43. Lücke-Hühle, C., Blakely, E. A., Ngo, F.Q.H., Chang, P. Y., and Tobias, C. A. Survival and kinetic response of V79 spheroids after exposure to heavy-ion beams. Submitted to Radiat. Res.

44. Rodriguez, A. and Alpen, E. L. Multicellular spheroid survival with accelerated heavy-ion beams. Submitted to Radiat. Res.

FUNDAMENTAL AND CLINICAL APPROACHES TO RADIORESISTANT CANCERS

.

© 1979, Elsevier/North-Holland Biomedical Press
Treatment of Radioresistant Cancers
M. Abe, K. Sakamoto and T.L. Phillips eds.

LOCAL CONTROL AND RADIATION DOSE OF SARCOMA OF SOFT TISSUE IN THE ADULT

HERMAN D. SUIT

Department of Radiation Medicine, Massachusetts General Hospital, Harvard

Medical School. Boston, MA 02114, U.S.A.

The sarcoma of soft tissue are classed as radiation resistant tumors.

There are in the literature a number of reports documenting that tumors in

this category may in fact be treated successfully by radiation alone. Based

on an experience in the treatment of more than 300 patients with sarcoma of

soft tissue my attitude is that tumors of this group may be managed by radia-

tion therapy alone with a reasonable likelihood of success provided: the

tumors are small or of moderate size, high radiation doses are employed

(equivalent of $\geq$7000 rad in 7 weeks given at 200 rads per fraction), that

modern equipment and sophisticated techniques are employed in order that

uninvolved tissue be excluded from the treatment volume to the maximum extent

feasible. Despite the success which can be achieved in the use of radiation

therapy alone, higher success rates and better functional results are

achievable with a combination of radiation therapy and surgery. The preferred

sequence is radiation therapy given pre-operatively and for slightly lesser

radiation dose levels ($\approx$6000 rad in 6 weeks) followed by conservative exci-

sional surgery.[1]

A substantial basis for the reputation of these lesions as being extra-

ordinarily radiation resistant is that in the early period of radiation therapy,

the relatively common presentation of the patient with sarcoma of soft tissue

was with a massive lesion. Equipment available during the 30's and 40's was

orthovoltage radiation and hence the central tumor dose was low in relationship

to the surface dose. That is, there was initial experience based on the use
of moderate radiation dose levels against large tumors. That success was not
common is hardly surprising. Nevertheless, occasional successes were achieved.
For example, Leucutia[2] (1935) presented results of the treatment of a patient
who had a recurrent fibrosarcoma in the scapular region who was alive and
well at 10 years after orthovoltage therapy alone. Cade[3] reviewed his experience in the management of a large series of patients with sarcoma of soft
tissue. Amongst his patients were 22 who for special reasons were not treated
by surgery but in fact received radiation alone. Of these 22 patients, 6 were
surviving free of evident tumor for 5-26 years. In 1966 Windeyer[4] and associates reported that 4 of 8 patients treated for fibrosarcoma by radiation
alone were free of local disease at more than 5 years. At the Memorial
Hospital in New York McNeer et al[5] reported an analysis of the results of the
treatment of 653 patients with sarcoma of soft tissue at that hospital. Of
these, 23 were treated by radiation therapy alone. Results are impressive in
that 14 of those 23 were reported as alive and well at 5 years and 8 of 20
were surviving at 10 years. Amongst 18 patients treated at the M.D. Anderson
Hospital to radiation doses in excess of 6300 rads, local control was achieved
in 14 (analysis as of August 1975, Suit, 1977[5] and 1979[6]). Actually of the 4
failures, one was a marginal miss. Some very long term disease free survivals
have been attained in that series. Of 11 patients who were Stage I or
Stage II, five are surviving with local control between 65 and 168 months.

At the Massachusetts General Hospital, radiation has been employed as the
sole treatment of 29 primary and recurrent sarcomas since 1970. The local
control data at one to seven years are presented in Table 1. As shown there
is a very strong relationship between radiation dose level and local control
frequency. Successful treatment of the primary lesion was infrequent at doses
corresponding to TDF values of less than 105 or approximate equivalent of

TABLE 1.

RADIATION DOSE LEVEL (TDF) AND LOCAL CONTROL OF SOFT TISSUE SARCOMA WHEN
TREATED BY RADIATION ALONE

Dose (TDF)	Tumor Size	<5	5-9	10-14	>15
≥105		2/2	4/9	2/2	2/3
95-104					0/1
80-94			1/3	0/1	0/3
<80			1/3	0/1	0/1

6500 rad delivered in daily treatments of 200 rad, 5 treatments per week.
Amongst this group of patients there was not an evident relationship between
local control frequency and tumor size. Although not shown, there were sub-
stantially higher dose levels employed in the largest tumors; namely, doses in
the range of 7000-8000 rad. Amongst those patients late tissue damage was un-
attractive. Nonetheless, a few patients can experience eradication of a large
primary tumor with acceptable levels of late tissue change.

As stated earlier our approach is combination of radiation therapy with surgery and that radiation therapy alone be employed only in those patients for
whom surgery is not feasible for technical reasons or the patient cannot accept
surgery for medical reasons or in special situations absolutely refuses to have
surgery.

Radiation Therapy Combined With Surgery.

Our success in the treatment of patients with large tumors by pre-operative
irradiation has been high. This is shown in Table 2. Here we see that of 15
patients who were treated by radiation therapy followed by excisional surgery,

TABLE 2

SARCOMA OF SOFT TISSUE TREATED BY RADIATION THERAPY FOLLOWED BY CONSERVATIVE RESECTION

Resection of Residual Mass

Stage	Local Control	Disease Free Survival
IB	3/3	3/3
IIB	4/4	4/4
IIIA	1/1	1/1
IIIB	7/7	4/7

Resection Attempted by not Completed

Stage	Local Control	Disease Free Survival
IIIB	1/2	0/2

local control has been obtained in all 15. In two patients resection was attempted but not completed and one of those has developed a local failure. This is a patient who had an extraosseous osteogenic sarcoma in the antecubital space. At the time of attempted excision the median nerve was observed to be completely surrounded by tumor and resection was not feasible. With the exception of one patient, a Stage IIIA, the patients treated by radiation therapy followed by surgery had large lesions; thus, these results are, for us, quite impressive. Our experience with patients seen after resectional surgery and treated post-operatively have also shown high frequency of local control. The experience amongst 58 patients treated by this manner are presented in Table 3 where we show local control as a function of size of tumor and dose level. For the total group, local control has been achieved in 50 of 58 patients or in 86% These data do not indicate strong dependency of local success on radiation dose. There were 20 of 22 local control among patients whose tumors were 5cm or less (91% local control rate) but for patients with tumors greater than 5cm

TABLE 3.

RADIATION DOSE LEVEL (TDF) AND LOCAL CONTROL OF SOFT TISSUE SARCOMA WHEN
TREATED BY EXCISION AND POST-OPERATIVE RADIATION THERAPY.

Dose (TDF)	Tumor Size (cm)				
	<5	5-9.9	10-14.9	≥15.0	
≥105	15/17	11/13	4/5	3/4	33/39
100-104.9	2/2	3/3	1/1	2/2	8/8
80-99.9	2/2	1/2		1/2	4/6
<80	1/1		2/2	2/2	5/5
	20/22	15/18	7/8	8/10	

the local success was 30 of 36 or 83%. Patients treated by the combined
modality has experienced a high local control rate. Importantly, very good
functional results are achieved in approximately 85% of the patients. That
is, there is no pain and no edema or if edema is present, is readily controlled by use of a jobst stocking.

Certainly, the dose levels which are referred to above are high, but for
permanent regression of large epithelial tumors (>5 cm) comparable dose
levels are required. This is true for squamous cell carcinomas and for
adenocarcinomas. I do not think that a convincing case can be made that the
tumors classed as sarcoma of soft tissue are more radiation resistant than
the adenocarcinomas and squamous cell carcinomas when the response to specified
radiation dose treatment schedules are assessed against tumors of comparable
sizes. Obviously, the sarcoma of soft tissue are quite resistant when compared with tumors in the lymphomas and seminoma category. A pertinent fact
is that many sarcomas of soft tissue are initially seen at the time that they
are much larger than 5 cm. A 5-10 cm diameter tumor in the head and neck
region, cervical region, breast, urinary bladder, uterine cervix, etc.,
would all be high stage and the clinician would expect that quite large
radiation doses would be employed if permanent control were anticipated.

REFERENCES

1. Suit, H.D. and Proppe, K.H. (1979) Sarcoma of Soft Tissue. In CANCER TREATMENT. K. Halnan, Ed. Chapman & Hall, Ltd. London, England. In Press.

2. Leucutia, T. (1935) Radiotherapy of sarcoma of the soft parts. Radiology 25:403-415.

3. Cade, S. (1951) Soft tissue tumours: their natural history and treatment. Section of surgery: president's address. Proc. Roy. Soc. Med. 44:19-36.

4. Windeyer, B., Dische, S. and Mansfield, C.M. (1966) The place of radiotherapy in the management of fibrosarcoma of the soft tissues. Clin. Radiol. 17:32-40.

5. McNeer, G.P., Cantin, J., Chu, F. and Nickson, J.J. (1968) Effectiveness of radiation therapy in management of sarcoma of soft somatic tissues. Cancer 22:391-397.

6. Suit, H.D. and Russell, W.O. (1977) Soft part tumors. Cancer 37:830-836.

7. Suit, H.D. and Proppe, K.H. (1979) Radiation therapy of soft tissue tumors. In Symposia: CHACON: XII International Cancer Congress, Buenos Aires, 1978. In Press.

© 1979, Elsevier/North-Holland Biomedical Press
Treatment of Radioresistant Cancers
M. Abe, K. Sakamoto and T.L. Phillips eds.

UNEVEN FRACTIONATION RADIOTHERAPY IN BRONCHOGENIC CARCINOMA

MASAJI TAKAHASHI, MITSUYUKI ABE, NARIYOSHI RI, YOSHIHIRO DODO,
SHIGEHARU DOKO and TAKEHIRO NISHIDAI
Department of Radiology, Faculty of Medicine, Kyoto University,
606, Kyoto (Japan)

INTRODUCTION

Despite the introduction of megavoltage radiation unit, little
significant increase in the cure rate of bronchogenic carcinoma
appears to have been achieved. The five year survival rates
published remain less than approximately 10% for locally advanced
inoperable bronchogenic carcinoma[1-5], and the results have not
been essentially improved for many years. It is considered,
therefore, that better results in survival rates for this disease
cannot be expected by conventional radiotherapy.

Recent advances in radiobiology have stimulated the development
of fractionation regimes based on scientific considerations instead of empiricism. Observations made during recent years with
a variety of biological materials suggest that the cellular repair
of sublethal radiation damage is an oxygen dependent, energy requiring process[6-9]. Therefore, oxygen is considered to have
sensitizing and at the same time restorative actions to radiation.
Révész[10] has demonstrated that the net oxygen effect on survival
will be product of the sensitizing and protective actions.
When the radiation dose is relatively small, the restorative action balances or even compensates for the sensitizing action.
On the other hand in the case of exposure to relatively large
doses, the extent of the recovery of oxically irradiated cells
will account for a smaller proportion of the cell lethality, and
the net survival for an oxic population will therefore decrease in
relation to that for an anoxic population of an identical size.
In addition, it has been demonstrated that a reoxygenation process
takes place in irradiated tumors[11-13]. From these experimental
results it is likely that after irradiation with a large dose,
e.g. 600 rad, the majority of the oxygenated cells will be killed
and the surviving tumor cells will constitute largely of hypoxic

194

or anoxic cells. Until the vascularization improves, little
oxygenation of the tumor can be expected. Therefore, large doses
may not be effective and a series of small dose fractions may be
of advantage. During this series of fractions, the anoxic tumor
cells will accumulate the radiation damage without recovery,
while normal tissues with the capacity to recover because of the
presence of oxygen, can be spared. When the vascularization
conditions are improved and reoxygenation is achieved, irradiation with a large dose, again followed by a series of small dose
fractions would appear to be a rational treatment schedule
(Fig. 1).

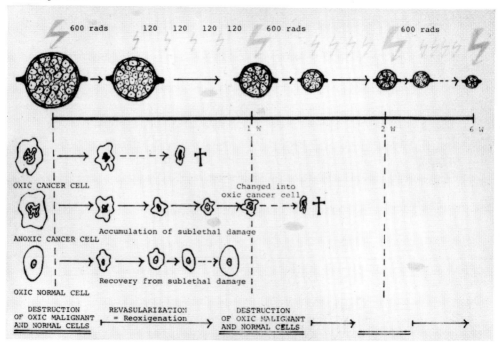

Fig. 1. Radiobiological basis of uneven fractionation radiotherapy.

MATERIAL

The material consisted of 132 consecutive patients, 120 out of
these patients were available for follow-up beyond more than 1
year. The patients were those who were diagnosed as inoperable
because of locally advanced stage or poor general condition. The
distribution of patients with regard to stage and histology was

shown in Tabs. 1 and 2 respectively. Staging of bronchogenic carcinoma was made according to the UICC classification proposed in 1978.

TABLE 1

STAGE DISTRIBUTION OF PATIENTS TREATED BY UNEVEN FRACTIONATION RADIOTHERAPY

Stage	No. of patients	Percent
I	9	7.5
II	37	30.8
III	58	48.3
IV	16	13.4
Total	120	100.0

TABLE 2

HISTOLOGICAL DISTRIBUTION OF PATIENTS TREATED BY UNEVEN FRACTIONATION RADIOTHERAPY

Histology	No. of patients	Percent
Squamous cell ca.	48	40.0
Adeno ca.	16	13.3
Undifferentiated cell ca.	12	10.0
Small cell ca.	6	5.0
Large cell ca.	6	5.0
Histologically unestablished, but cytologically malignant	32	26.7
Total	120	100.0

METHODS

All patients were treated by a ^{60}Co unit with one ventral and one dorsal opposing fields. In general, the primary lesion and the regional lymph nodes were treated with margins of at least 2 cm in excess of those necessary for the volume believed to contain the cancer. The treatment scheme used in this trial is illustrated in Fig. 2.

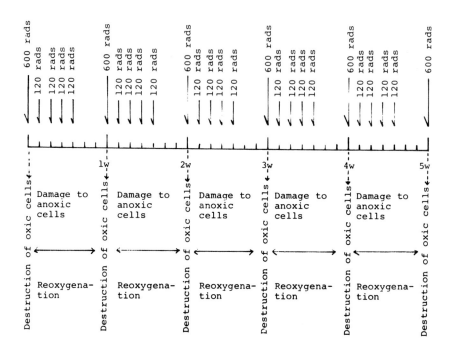

Fig. 2. Schedule of uneven fractionation radiotherapy.

Treatment was started with a dose of 600 rad which is expected
to eliminate a great majority of oxic tumor cells. The residual
tumor cells are considered to belong, in most part, to an anoxic
component. As a subsequent treatment, 120 rad daily doses were
given 4 times with an attempt to let the anoxic cells accumulate
radiation damage and exposure the normal oxic cells to a small
injury. No treatments were made on Saturday and Sunday. After
the series of irradiation with low doses which is expected to
lead reoxygenation of the tumor, a second large dose exposure
with 600 rad was given, followed by daily treatment with small
doses until a total dose of 6,000 rad was delivered.

RESULTS
Crude survival rates of patients treated by uneven fractionation radiotherapy was shown in Tab. 3.

TABLE 3

CRUDE SURVIVAL RATES OF PATIENTS TREATED BY UNEVEN FRACTIONATION
RADIOTHERAPY

Year	No. of patients	Patients alive	Crude survival rate
1	120	43	35.8
2	101	17	16.8
3	68	9	13.2
4	45	3	6.7
5	23	3	13.0

The 3 and 5 year crude survival rates were 13.2% and 13.0%
respectively.

DISCUSSION

In order to examine the effectiveness of the uneven fractionation radiotherapy, we made a preliminary comparison of the
results with those obtained by conventional radiotherapy in
earlier years. During the years 1962 to 1974, 314 patients with
bronchogenic carcinoma were treated by radiation alone in Kyoto
University Hospital. The patients were those who were deemed
inoperable by the thoracic surgeon because of locally advanced
stage or poor general condition. Of 314 patients, 80 had to be
eliminated from the final evaluation because of the presence of
distant metastases at the onset of treatment or because the
patient was unable to receive at least 4,000 rad of a total tumor
dose. Nine patients were not included in this study because,
although they had complete radiotherapy, the follow-up is incomplete or missing. Thus of the 314 patients 89 were not
eligible for this study. The remaining 225 patients were
reviewed.

The distribution of patients according to stage and histology
was shown in Tabs. 4 and 5, respectively. All patients were
treated with ^{60}Co unit with parallel opposing fields. Irradiation was administered with 5 fractions a week with a daily dose
of 150 to 200 rad, with a tumor dose of 4,000 to 7,000 rad over
4 - 8 weeks. The crude survival rates of patients treated by
conventional radiotherapy was shown in Tab. 6.

TABLE 4

STAGE DISTRIBUTION OF PATIENTS TREATED BY CONVENTIONAL
RADIOTHERAPY

Stage	No. of patients	Percent
I	7	3.1
II	133	59.1
III	61	27.1
IV	24	10.7
Total	225	100.0

TABLE 5

HISTOLOGICAL DISTRIBUTION OF PATIENTS TREATED BY CONVENTIONAL
RADIOTHERAPY

Histology	No. of patients	Percent
Squamous cell ca.	61	27.1
Adeno ca.	34	15.1
Undifferentiated cell ca.	35	15.6
Small cell ca.	9	4.0
Histologically unestablished, but cytologically malignant	86	38.2
Total	225	100.0

TABLE 6

CRUDE SURVIVAL RATES OF PATIENTS TREATED BY CONVENTIONAL
RADIOTHERAPY

Year	No. of patients	Patients alive	Crude survival rate
1	225	62	27.5
2	218	27	12.3
3	199	9	4.5
4	186	6	3.2
5	175	6	3.4

In order to analyze the results obtained by uneven fractionation radiotherapy, comparison was made of stage as well as
histological distribution and the crude survival rates between
two treatment modalities. Fig. 3 shows the stage distribution in
uneven fractionation radiotherapy and conventional radiotherapy
groups. Fig. 4 demonstrates the histological distribution in both
groups. The crude survival rate in both groups was illustrated in
Fig. 5. At each observation year, the survival rate is higher in
uneven fractionation group than that in conventional group by
about 4 to 10%, despite the fact the proportion of advanced cases
was somewhat larger in uneven fractionation group. The number of
patients treated by uneven fractionation radiotherapy are not
enough to afford any definitive evaluation, but the results obtained so far seem most encouraging.

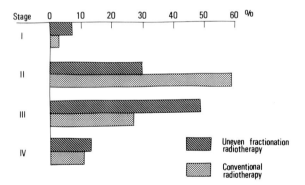

Fig. 3. Stage distribution of patients treated by uneven fractionation radiotherapy and conventional radiotherapy.

200

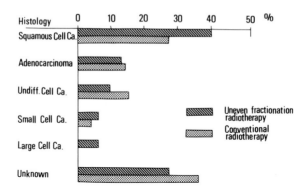

Fig. 4. Histological distribution of patients treated by uneven fractionation radiotherapy and conventional radiotherapy.

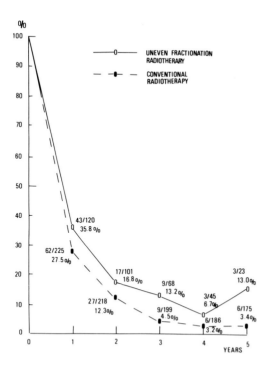

Fig. 5. Crude survival rates of patients treated by uneven fractionation radiotherapy and conventional radiotherapy.

The efficacy of uneven fractionation irradiation on the tumor
was examined by the measurement of the tumor regression rate.
It was calculated from the measurement of the tumor size in the
chest X-ray film. The product of the two diameters was used as
an indicator of the tumor size. The number of cases in which the
tumor size could be measured was 22 in the uneven fractionation
group. For comparison with patients treated with this new
regime, 13 conventionally treated patients were selected in considering identical anatomic site, clinical stage and histology of
the tumor. The histological distribution in both groups which
may play the most significant role in determining the tumor
regression by irradiation was illustrated in Fig. 6. The distribution is heavily weighed with squamous cell carcinoma in each
group. Fig. 7 demonstrates the tumor regression curves in both
groups.

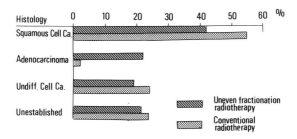

Fig. 6. Histological distribution in uneven fractionation
radiotherapy and conventional radiotherapy groups.

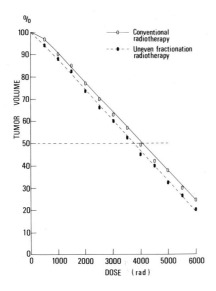

Fig. 7. Tumor regression curves in uneven fractionation radiotherapy and conventional radiotherapy groups.

The 50% tumor regression dose (TRD_{50}) which would be necessary to regress the tumor of its half volume was estimated from Fig. 7. The TRD_{50} for conventional radiotherapy group and uneven fractionation radiotherapy group were 4,000 and 3,700 rad respectively. No significant difference was observed in both groups.

Then, the degree of damage to normal pulmonary tissue induced by uneven fractionation radiotherapy and by conventional radiotherapy was compared using radiation fibrosis as the measure of response. For comparison, patients in both groups were selected in considering identical radiation doses and field sizes. According to the density of the shadow appeared in the chest X-ray film, the degree of radiation fibrosis was classified as F_3 (the density is almost equal to that of the liver shadow), F_2 (almost equal to that of the rib shadow) and F_1 (lower than that of the rib shadow).

Tab. 7 shows the comparison of the degree of radiation fibrosis induced by both treatment modalities. Estimation of lung fibrosis in chest X-ray films was made four months after completion of radiotherapy.

TABLE 7

GRADE OF PULMONARY FIBROSIS INDUCED BY RADIOTHERAPY AND ITS
INCIDENCE IN RELATION TO THE MODE OF TREATMENT

Grade of fibrosis	Uneven fractionation radiotherapy	Conventional radiotherapy
F_1	11/42 (26.2%)	5/26 (19.2%)
F_2	19/42 (45.2%)	9/26 (34.6%)
F_3	12/42 (28.6%)	12/26 (46.2%)

As is clear in Tab. 7, radiation fibrosis of the lung was found
to be more prominent in conventional group than uneven fractionation group. The advantage of uneven fractionation radiotherapy
over conventional radiotherapy in diminishing damage to normal
tissues agrees well with other observations[14]. The characteristic
of uneven fractionation irradiation is less pronounced damage to
normal structures and can possibly be attributed to facilitate
recovery of normal cells from sublethal damage during a series of
small dose fractions. The decreased damage to normal tissues
surrounding the tumor is considered to be favorable to the control
of tumors by a more efficient local sterilization of radiation
damaged neoplastic cells.

Although final evaluation has to await the accumulation of
further experience, the results obtained so far encourage the
continuation of uneven fractionation radiotherapy.

CONCLUSIONS

Uneven fractionation radiotherapy based upon radiobiological
considerations has been introduced in the treatment of bronchogenic carcinoma. The efficacy of the method was analyzed in relation
to the results obtained by conventional radiotherapy. The crude
survival rates were higher in uneven fractionation radiotherapy
group than that in conventional radiotherapy group by about 4 to
10% at each observation year.

Radiation fibrosis of the lung was found to be less prominent
in uneven fractionation radiotherapy group than conventional
radiotherapy group.

The results obtained so far seem most encouraging.

ACKNOWLEDGEMENTS

We wish to thank Prof. L. Révész Karolinska Institute for his excellent suggestions to our uneven fractionation scheme.

This work was supported by a Cancer Research Grant from the Ministry of Welfare, Japan.

REFERENCES

1. Deeley, T.J. and Singh, S.P. (1967) Thorax, 22, 562-566.
2. Eichhorn, H.J. and Lessel, A. (1968) Strahlentherapie, 136, 411-413.
3. Morrison, R. and Deeley, T.J. (1969) Lancet II, 618-620.
4. Schnepper, E.H. (1967) Strahlentherapie, 133, 176-183.
5. Abe, M. et al. (1976) J. Jap. Soc. Cancer Ther. 11, 23-35.
6. Belli, J.A. et al. (1967) J. nat. Cancer Inst. 38, 673-682.
7. Hall, H.J. (1972) Radiat. Res. 49, 405-415.
8. Littbrand, B. and Révész, L. (1969) Brit. J. Radiol. 42, 914-924.
9. Suit, H. and Urano, M. (1969) Radiat. Res. 37, 423-434.
10. Révész, L. (1973) Fraction size in radiobiology and radiotherapy, Igakushoin, Tokyo, pp. 142-155.
11. Howes, A.E. (1969) Brit. J. Radiol. 42, 441-447.
12. Kallman, R.F. et al. (1970) J. nat. Cancer Inst. 44, 369-377.
13. Rubin, P.P. and Casarett, G. (1966) Clin. Radiol. 17, 346-355.
14. Siracká, E. et al. (1971) Neoplasma, 18, 607-616.

© 1979, Elsevier/North-Holland Biomedical Press
Treatment of Radioresistant Cancers
M. Abe, K. Sakamoto and T.L. Phillips eds.

THE PLACE OF COMBINED TREATMENT WITH BLEOMYCIN AND RADIATION

YASUSHI SHIGEMATSU and YOSHIHIRO TANAKA
Department of Radiology, Osaka University Medical School, Osaka, JAPAN 553

INTRODUCTION

For a long time, combined use of chemical drugs with radiation has been tried widely in the world, to improve the tumor control rate and the survival figure. However, very few have been recognized to be really beneficial in clinical practice, inspite of hopeful description in a fundamental and preliminary stage of the study.

Considering the study on the combined use of Bleomycin and radiation for the past several years at the department, there have been three steps the authors would like to divide it into as follows : 1) preliminary study (1972-1974), 2) co-operative controlled trial (1974-1976) and 3) analysis of 181 intra-oral carcinomas at the department (1972-1978) for this presentation. At the department, the phase 1 study was not got in touch with, and a high dose of the drug was rarely applied because of the high risk of pulmonary complication. The study was started on an occasion when an advanced carcinoma of the lower gum was beutifully controlled with a combination of rather small doses of radiation and Bleomycin.

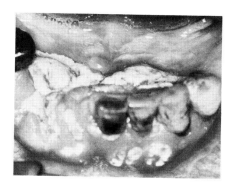 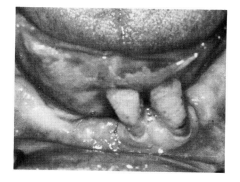

November 24, 1972

November 13, 1973
(1 year afer RT+BLM)

Fig. 1. A case of carcinoma of the lower gum controlled by combined treatment with radiotherapy and Bleomycin

PRELIMINARY STUDY (1972-1974)

The above mentioned case is presented in Figure 1. This is a case of squamous cell carcinoma of the lower gum, in a 60 year old man. In November 1972, this was treated with radiation and Bleomycin. On a three times weekly schedule, a total of 2700 rad delivered in 3 weeks. Bleomycin was started 2 weeks before the start of radiotherapy and the total of Bleomycin was 105 mg. The left side picture shows the local condition before the treatment, and the right sided is the one one year afer the treatment. All of the teath dropped out by the last follow-up on April 20, 1979, the patient has been doing well without any problem in the mandible.

Such cases of preliminary trial were accumulated from October 1972 through May 1974, and a total of 39 intra-oral carcinomas were examined. Special attention was paid to the advanced carcinoma of the lower gum, since this disease had been difficult to control by radiation alone without developping bone necrosis. The employed treatment schedule consisted of two parts : the initial treatment was the trial of the combined therapy with radiation and Bleomycin, and the subsequent treatment if necessary was individualized by case, such as operation or further radiotherapy. Howerer, in the beginning days of the trial, patient was often managed by surgery to emamine the specimen. The result was already published by Tanaka et al,[1] and the minimum required dose to control such tumors was found to be a combination of 1200 ret by radiation and 60-70 mg of Bleomycin, or 1100 ret of radiation and 90-105 mg of Bleomycin. This dose schedule also incicated the tolerance limit of mucosal membrane in most of the cases.

CO-OPERATIVE STUDY (1974-1976)

Encouraged by the preliminary study, a co-operative trial was planned in 1974 with Kimura at Kobe University and Abe at Kyoto University. Eighteen institution of Kansai district (Kyoto-Osaka-Kobe area) joined this study. In addition to the intra-oral carcinoma, bronchogenic and esophageal carcinoma were decided to examine. Kimura was engaged in bronchogenic carcinoma, Abe in esophageal carcinoma and the author took care of the intra-oral carcinoma.

The study was started in September 1974 and discontinued in June 1976. During the period, 50 patients with bronchogenic carcinoma, 72 patients with esophageal carcinoma and 67 patients with intra-oral carcinoma were enrolled in this study.

The patient was randomized into two fixed schedule for the first step : Option 1, 3000 rad in 3 weeks RT and 90 mg Bleomycin (15 mg x 6, twice weekly), Option 2, 3000 rad in 3 weeks RT only. After the judgment of early effect two weeks later, patient was assigned to subsequent treatment program, which was considered best by the participating doctors. The study could thus proceed without ethical problems. At any rate, a dose of 3000 rad in 3 weeks used for the initial treatment in the control group (option 1) is much lower than the curative dose level, and the subsequent treatment must very much influence the final result. Incidentally, a number of cases which were considered candidates for radical radiotherapy received a total dose of 6000-7000 rad, using something like split-course technique in the radiotherapy alone group.

Concerning the cases of bronchogenic and esophageal carcinomas, Abe[2] summarized the data in 1977, and following conclusions were drawn.

1) In bronchogenic carcinomas, no significant difference was observed in tumor regression or survival rate between both groups.

2) In esophageal carcinoma, Bleomycin in combination with radiation markedly improved the regresion rate of polypoid type tumor, while no significant improvement was observed in other types, such as funnel or spiral. The survival rate didn't show any significant difference between combined and radiation alone group.

In the intra-oral carcinomas, which was analysed by the authors in 1977, there was a variety of site and stage, and it was difficult to discuss the material in total. The case distribution is shown in Table 1.

TABLE 1
CASE DISTRIBUTION OF CO-OPERATIVE RT-BLM TRIAL IN INTRA-ORAL CARCINOMA, 1974-1976

	Tongue	Mouth Floor	Lower Gum	Upper Gum	Hard Palate	Cheek	Total
RT+BLM	5	6	12	1	5	2	31
RT only	6	3	13	5	1	2	30

TABLE 2
SURVIVAL RATE OF PATIENTS WITH LOWER GUM CARCINOMA, CO-OPERATIVE RT-BLM TRIAL SERIES, 1974-1976

	0.5yr	1.0	1.5	2.0
RT+BLM	12(5)/12	12(3)/12	11(3)/11	8(3)/8
RT only	12(2)/12	11(2)/12	8(2)/10	4(1)/6

( ) : Controlled with Initial RT only

When the cases of carcinoma of the lower gum were examined, there were some-what higher local control rate and survival rate in BLM-RT group (Table 2).

However, the case distribution wasn't uniform in the two groups. More local-ly advanced cases are found in the control group than in the BLM-RT combined group as is shown in Table 3, and any conclusive comment could not be drawn from these material. The authors returned back to the analysis of the own material as Osaka University Hospital.

TABLE 3

CASE DISTRIBUTION OF CARCINOMA OF THE LOWER GUM BY TNM-CLASSIFICATION, CO-OPERATIVE RT-BLM TRIAL SERIES, 1974-1976.

	RT + BLM				RT only	
	T2	T3			T2	T3
N0	5	1		N0	2	4
N1	2	2		N1	3	3
N2	1	1		N2	0	0

ANALYSIS OF 181 INTRA-ORAL CARCINOMAS AT THE DEPARTMENT

For the past 8 years, there have been 181 patients with intra-oral carcinomas initially treated with combined treatment with Bleomycin and radiation.

TABLE 4

CASE DISTRIBUTION AND TREATMENT MODALILITY IN 181 INTRA-ORAL CARCINOMAS INITIALLY TREATED BLEOMYCIN AND RADIATION.

	No of cases	Subsequent Treatment				
			Surgery		Radiotherapy	
		none	primary	Neck	Brachy	External
Lower gum	60	11	37	17	1	11(7)
Upper gum	25	4	16	6	1	5(1)
Cheek	24	8	4	2	8	9(2)
Tongue	32	—	5	8	14	5(2)
Mouth Floor	36	1	13	12	13	10(4)
Palate	4	—	2	1	—	2
Total	181	24	77	46	37	42

( ) : combined treatment with RT+BLM repeated.

Table 4 shows the number of cases by site and the treatment modality including individualized subsequent treatment. Although the tongue is the most common
site of intra-oral carcinomas and there have been over 50 cases annually regist-
ered at the department, this was not allocated to the study as far as the case
was treatable with interstitial radiotherapy, since there was another program
for the disease.

Of 60 patients with carcinoma of the lower gum, forty patients were followed
over 2 years, and local control rate and survival rate are shown in Table 5,
according to TNM classification by UICC, 1973.

TABLE 5

TWO YEAR CONTROL RATE OF CARCINOMA OF THE LOWER GUM, BLM+RT, OSAKA UNIVERSITY
HOSPITAL, 1972-1978

	T1	T2	T3	Total
N0	(1) 2/3	(3) 7/9	(1) 4/6	(5) 13/18
N1	—	(3) 9/10	5/6	(3) 14/16
N2	—	(1) 1/1	(1) 2/2	(1) 3/3
N3			0/3	(0) (0)/3
	(1) 2/3	(6) 17/20	(2) 11/17	(9) 30/40

( ) : Patients controlled by initial RT + BLM

The number in parenthesis indicates the cases controlled by initial combined
treatment alone, and the total number of numerator indicates the one including
the cases salvaged by subsequent treatment. Of 23 cases of T1 and T2, seven
remain controlled, i.e., 30% with initial treatment alone ; whereas only 2 cases
were controlled of 17 cases of T3, i.e., approximately 10%. More than half of
the failure cases by initial treatment was salvaged by subsequently performed
surgery, and thirty of 40 patients have been doing well without recurrence, when
such cases are included.

By the way, another parameter to evaluate the possibility of local control
must be the grade of bony destruction of the mandible. This is usually devided
into 3 categories : erosive, permeative and moth-eaten in the x-ray findings.

As shown in Table 6, more than half of 37 cases having erosive or permeative
findings, were controlled by initial treatment, whereas only 2 cases, out of 13
cases with moth-eaten findings were controlled. Althouth the tumor out-look
such as exophytic or infiltrative is another paramenter, the difference by this
is not so remarkable as the one by T-classification and the grade of bony destruction.

TABLE 6

TUMOR DISAPPEARANCE RATE OF CARCINOMA OF THE LOWER GUM, BLM+RT, OSAKA
UNIVERSITY HOSPITAL, 1972-1978

	Tumor Disappearance Rate		
By X-ray Findings of Mandible	erosive	permeative	moth-eaten
	12/21 (57%)	9/16 (56%)	2/13 (15%)
By Tumor Outlook	superficial exophytic nodular	infiltrative ulcerative	
	11/19 (58%)	12/35 (34%)	

In figure 2, the cummulative rates of local control and survival of the carcinoma of the lower gum are shown. The broken line in the middle, in which the cases of no malignant cells in the surgical specimen were added, could be the possible local control rate by initial treatment of combined modality with approximentaly 3000 rad and 100 my Bleomycin.

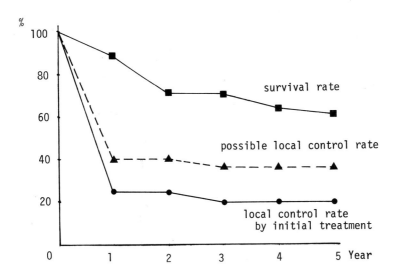

Fig. 2. Cummulative local control rate and survival rate of patients with carcinoma of the lower gum, RT+BLM Series, Osaka University Hospital, 1972-1978

The experience of combined treatment with Bleomycin and radiation for carcinoma of the lower gum at the department is summarized as follows:

1) A minimum required dose for local control of the disease, could be a combination of 3000 rad of radiation in 3 weeks and 100 mg of Bleomycin during the period.

2) For the treatment, the side effect as limiting factor is the mucositis, and none of the cases of the series developed pulmonary complication.

3) The tumor control rate is influenced by the tumor size and the grade of bony destruction of the mandible.

4) In the cases controlled by initial combined treatment, no one developed troubles of the mandible, in the follow-up study for the past 8 years.

DISCUSSION

There have been a variety of discussions on the mechanism of Bleomycin to control the tumor cells. Considering the combined effect of Bleomycin with radiation, most discussions seem to have been directed to a point whether it is additive effect or sensitizing. However, considering the material of carcinoma of the lower gum in this series, the difference of concentration of the drug to the tissue seems to be a more important factor. The authors looked for the past fundamental data of relative concentration of the drug in different tissues and there was one by Umezawa et al[3]., in which a low concentration to the bone is shown (Table 7). This could be a help in interpreting the result of the present series.

At any rate, the survival rate has also improved as high as 60% in 5 years in this series.

Since the medical background isn't the same as the historical control, the authors wouldn't like to have any comment on the matter at this moment. However, it can be stressed that the program above

TABLE 7

DISTRIBUTION OF ^{3}H-BLEOMYCIN AMONG ORGANS OF THE MICE 1HR. AFTER SUBCUT. INJ

	Bleomycin (mcg)/g of organ
Liver	8.5
Spleen	4.2
Kidney	47.6
Urinary Bladder	78.7
Small Intestion	13.5
Lung	15.8
Tongue	8.5
Skin	13.3
Bone	3.6
Muscle	8.5
Peritoneum	28.5

by Umezawa et al, 1968

mentioned has become routine in our slinical practice with asfety on an out patient base, and the patients controlled by the initial combined treatment have been enjoying better life than the patients in the past.

REFERENCES

1. Tanaka, Y. et al. (1976) Int. J. Radiation Oncology Biol. Phys., 1, 1189-1193.

2. Abe, M. et al. (1978) Recent Results in Cancer Research, 63, Springer-Verlag/Berlin-Heidelberg-New York, pp. 169-178.

3. Umezawa, H. et al. (1968) J. Antibiotics, 21, 638-642.

© 1979, Elsevier/North-Holland Biomedical Press
Treatment of Radioresistant Cancers
M. Abe, K. Sakamoto and T.L. Phillips eds.

CONSTRUCTION OF BLOOD VESSELS OF EXPERIMENTAL TUMORS - SOME CONSIDERATIONS
ON THE RADIORESISTANCY -

JUN EGAWA, KUNIAKI ISHIOKA
Department of Radiology, Teikyo University School of Medicine,
Kaga, Itabashi, Tokyo 173 (Japan)

INTRODUCTION

The vascular structure of tumors was widely investigated and reported by
many authors. The knowledge of the construction of microvascualr system and
microcirculation would be important for the understanding of the radiosensitivity of tumors, and might be applied to the radiotherapy of tumors. There are
several techniques for the observation of vascular structure of experimental
tumors. We used scanning electron microscope for the observation of capillary
cast, the very fine details can be visualized although the correlation of
capillary to the surrounding tissue can not be examined. In this paper, vascular
structures and effect of radiation on several transplanted tumors were reported.

TECHNIQUE OF EXAMINATION

Some of the techniques for observation of vascular system can be classified
as follows: the first group is that the injection of some materials is made
under almost physiological pressure, then the tissue is fixed and thick section
is made, then observed under microscope[1,2,3]. As for the injected materials,
Carbon-Gelatin, India-Ink-Gelatin, India-Ink, Lead Oxide, Silver Nitrate and
radiopaque substances are used. The ideal injected material might be physically
and chemically capable of permeating the finest vascular channels without
agglutinating. The observation of the structure are almost two dimensional
because the section of tissue was made, therefore the relationships of capillary
to the surrounding tissue can be investigated. The second type of examination
is microangiography, here radiopaque substance such as Barium Sulfate or iodide
contrast media is injected and radiographed with soft X-ray[4,5,6,7]. Overall
view of capillary might be visualized. The third one which we used is resin
cast method, which was reported in 1950 by Batson[8]. In 1971, Murakami[9] reported
scanning electron micrographs of some of the capillary meshes of the rat repro-
duced by a corrosion cast technique. By the technical improvement, he showed
beautiful photographs. Because of the very fine detailes of the capillary was
demonstrated, we applied it to the study of microvasculature of some of abdominal organs[10], experimental tumors[11] and the effect of radiation or anti-cancer

drug of them.

Technical details of resin cast method.

Preparation of resin. The base of resin was methyl-methacrylate monomer. Before injection, the resin had to be freshly prepared. First, 2.4-dichloro-benzoyl peroxide was added to the monomer up to a final concentration of 2 per cent. The mixture was then warmed to about 75°C and thereafter rapidly cooled. Then benzoyl peroxide was added, and just before th injection into the animal, N,N- dimethylanilin up to 2 per cent.

Resin injection and corrosion casting. The animals were anesthetized with ethylether and decapitated, and then irrigated with Ringer solution through the aorta. The prepared mixture was injected into the thoracic aorta under moderate pressure. The injected animals were placed in hot water (60-70°C) and kept at about 70°C in an incubator. After a few hours, Sodium Hydroxide (about 20%) was added for corrosion of the soft tissues. The resin cast obtained were washed and dried with ethyl alcohol in air. Resin cast is shown in Fig. 1. The tumor is visualized at the lateral side of upper thigh.

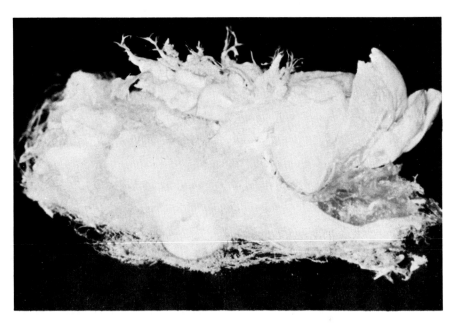

Fig. 1. Resin cast of blood vessels of a mouse.

Scanning electron microscopy   The dried whole body resin cast was dissected. The resin cast were fixed on an alminium block with a silver paste, and then exposed to vacuum evaporation with carbon and gold. These casts, which were coated by electron dense materials, were examined and photographed with a scanning electron microscope (Model MSM-4, Hitachi, Japan).

The characteristics of resin cast method are summarized as follows. As for the advantage of this method, at first, three dimensional observation is possible, second, interesting part of capillary mesh can be visualized by dissection, and arterial system, capillary and venous system can be demonstrated. As the side of disadvantage, because resin is injected by hand pressure, the physiological condition might be destroyed. The second important disadvantage is that the tissue are disolved by Sodium Hydroxide, so the correlation of the capillary to the surrounding tissue is entirely lost.

We tried to measure capillary width and intercapillary distance. Magnification is defined at the fixed plane of the sample, so the real magnification at the other part of the sample was not obtained. Then the measurement of intercapillary distance is too much complicated. Up to now, we can not still describe it with some accuracy.

VASCULAR CONSTRUCTION OF EXPERIMENTAL TUMORS

For this experiment, we used four kind of transplanted tumors, those are squamous cell carcinoma (pubic tumor, kindly supplied by Dr.Sakamoto), Ehrlich ascites carcinoma, ascites hepatoma AH 109A, AH 7974. Ninety mice and rats were used. At 5 to 15 days after transplantation of cells into the bilateral subcutaneous tissue of rump, tumors measured 2.5 to 15 mm in diameter were served for experiment.

The vascular construction of the four tumors was very similar. The main features of the capillaries of tumors were irregularity, tortuousity, sinusoid-like and tapering. The vascularity was complicated. But the appearances of the capillary network had a similar topographic position within the tumors, this is illustrated schematically in Fig. 2. In small tumors, extruding capillaries in the surface of the tumor mass were branched from larger vessels. The terminals were not connected with other exterior vessels. This capillary seems to invade radially from the tumor surface into the surrounding tissue. As shown in Fig. 3. , blood vessels with a wave-like apparance running parallel to each other were lying deeper on the mass (Fig. 4.). In the next inner layer, sinusoid-like (Fig. 5.) and tortous vessels (Fig. 6.) were observed. In a further layer, located near the central necrotic cavity, the capillaries ran

216

The schema of tumour vascular construction

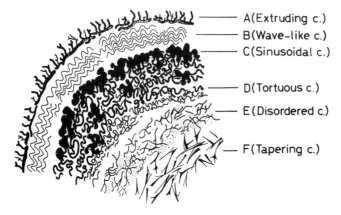

A(Extruding c.)
B(Wave-like c.)
C(Sinusoidal c.)

D(Tortuous c.)

E(Disordered c.)

F(Tapering c.)

Fig. 2.

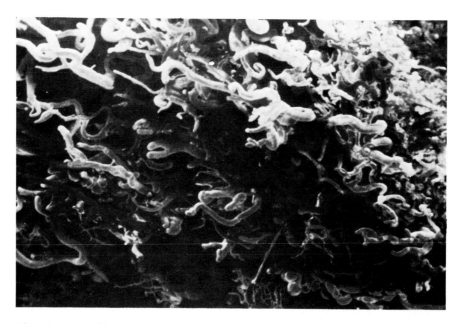

Fig. 3. Extruding capillaries on the surface of tumor mass.

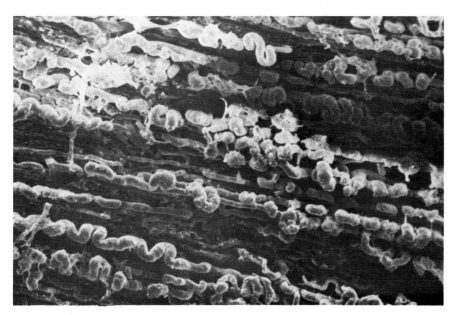

Fig. 4. Wave-like capillaries.

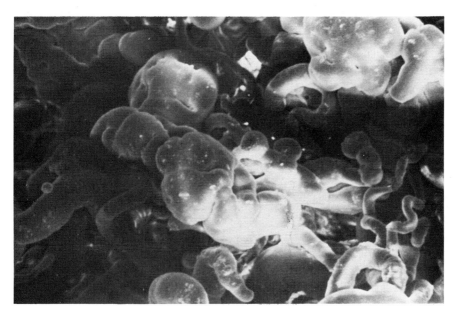

Fig . 5. Sinusoid like capillaries.

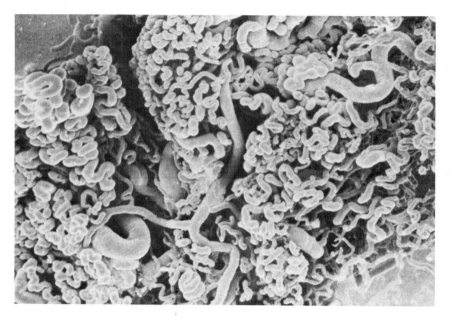

Fig. 6.   Tortuous vessels.

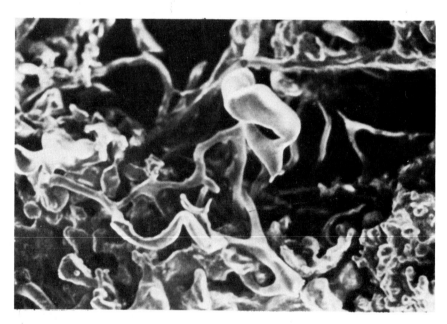

Fig. 7.Disorderly running capillaries.

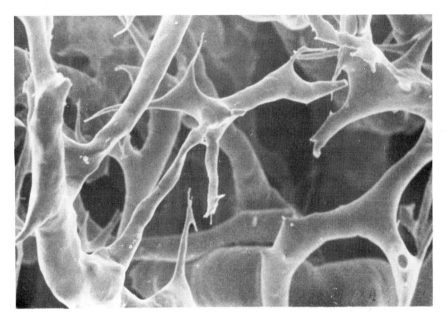

Fig. 8. Tapering capillaries in the central necrotic area.

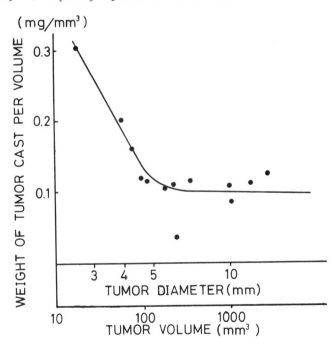

Fig. 9. Correlation between tumor volume and weight of the vascular cast per volume unit.

in disordered fashion (Fig. 7.). The vessels were irregular, regardless if
they were considered to be degenerated or destructed. Leakage of the resin
was often observed in this layer. In the central necrotic cavity, tapering
capillaries existed (Fig. 8.). The vascular structure was not changed significantly when the tumor size was between 5 to 15 mm diameter, but in tumors
with a diameter less than 3 mm, the tapering blood vessels which were found in
and around the necrotic cavity, were not observed. These small tumors mainly
contained tortuous and sinusoid-like vessels.

Quantitative analysis of weight of vascualr cast and tumor volume was made.
As shown in Fig. 9. , when the tumor volume (length X width X thickness) was
less than about 125 mm^3, the density of the vascualr cast was inversely
proportional to the tumor volume, when it was more than 125 mm^3, the density
was not correlated to tumor volume. This might be due to the developement
of necrosis in tumors.

Our findings of vascular structure can be compared to other authors. We
did not find much differences. Kawamura[12] described when tumor grew to 1 cm
in diameter, fine vascular networks were seen surrounding a central necrotic
area. The capillaries were fairly regular and uniform diameter, as the tumor
grew to 2 cm in diameter, the vascular bed of the tumor became more irregular
and many vascular areas are observed in the ntwork where necrosis gradually
developed. McAlister[13] described the specific and characteristic vascular
pattern regardless of tumour size. Saeki[14] examined C3H mouse mammary carcinoma, vascularization of non treated tumors, of recurrent tumors and of tumors
transplanted into a previously X-irradiated tumor bed was examined microangio-
graphically. In the non treated tumor, vascularization was peripheral with
penetrating vessels. Rich vascularization was located only in the periphery
where abundant fine vessels branched, but never stretched into a tumor center.
Rubin[15] described the three kind of vascular patterns, our tumor corresponded
to the one of them. Important findings of vascular structure of human gastric
cancer was reported by Maruyama, National Cancer Center Hospital in Tokyo. He
examined capillary system of it and classified the patterns in 6 groups, and
correlated with histology. A bundel shaped vessels are rich in differentiated
carcinoma, waving vessels are in differentiated carcinoma with microcirculatory
disturbance, reticular vessels are rich in undifferentiated carcinoma, laking
vessels are found in stromal vessels and in muconodular carcinoma, dwarf tree
shaped vessels are found in stromal vessels in infiltrative carcinoma, and
coiling vessels are found as a submucosal veacular proliferation in scirrhous
carcinoma. Foundamental patterns which is seen in experimental tumors would be

very much similar to that of human gastric cancer.

When the tumor grows, expansion to the surrounding tissue progresses and also necrotic cavity in the center formed. The extruding club-like capillaries on the surface of tumors were recognized[16]. The presence of these capillaries could be closely related to the tumor growth and also to the invasion of the tumor into surrounding tissue. The tapering capillaries ocurring in and around necrotic cavities seems to be regressively changed vessels. They may originally have been tortous vessels. As the necrosis increases, their diameter will become more and more irregular, probably ending in a tapering shape. With further degeneration of the capillaries a necrotic cavity is formend. Yamaura[17] reported tumor vasculature developed in rats ascites hepatoma AH 109A tissue transplanted into the rat transparent chamber. He divided the tumor vessel growth into 4 stages acording to the changes in vascular morphology. Stage I is slight capillary alterations, stage II is formation of fine capillary networks and change in veins, stage III is the modifications in arteries and stage IV is necrosis. The outer layer of the tumors remained in stage I,II, even a necrosis was started at the center.

We did not work much about morphometric study but as shown in Fig. 9. At the time of onset of necrosis, the curve become rather constant. Hilmas[18] reported the relation between vascular volume, vessel diameter, vessel length, surface area and necrotic tissue volume in C3H/Bi mammary carcinoma during tumor growth. The vascular volume did not change significantly during tumor growth but remained a relatively constant proportion of the total viable tumor volume. However necrotic tissue volume increased suddenly when a certain tumor volume was reached and then increased only slowly.

As a summary of our study of vascular structure of experimental tumors, we propose six patterns of capillary which is located in almost identical position in the tumor.

RADIATION EFFECT ON THE VASCULAR STRUCTURE OF EXPERIMENTAL TUMORS

The effect of radiation on capillary of tumors can be divided into morphological changes and functional one. Small blood vessels will be damaged as a direct effect of irradiation, early and late changes will be observed. Vascular structure of tumors is also effected secondary to the damage of tumor cells. Probably fuctional changes are predominate in early stage, but vascualr construction and vascular patterns will be modified in a few days. Reinhold[19] examined the radiation damage of capillary endothelium, he obtained 170 rad as for D_0, 7 as a extrapolation number, and 340 rad as for D_q. Epithelial cell has almost same radiosensitivity as the supporting cells. The many works were done about the functional change of capillary by irradiation (Hilmas[18], Saeki[14], Song[20], Clement[21], Pochen[22], Fujiwara[23], Tannok[24], Moss[25], Reinhold[26]).

Hilmas described the morphological changes after irradiation. There was a transit disappearance of the more variable shaped, sinusoid-type vessels, and the appearance of improved filling with increased numbers of smaller diameter vessels. The most interesting problems will be whether vascular construction will change or not by irradiation. Acording to the shrinkage of tumors, capillary mesh became dense (Rubin[15]).

We examined the effect of radiation on the blood capillary of Ehrlich ascites carcinoma of 54 mice. At 14 days after transplantation of tumor cells, when the size of transplanted solid tumor was about 10 to 12 mm in diameter, 30 Gy of a telecobalt gamma rays were given. At 1, 3, 5, 10, 20 and 30 days after irradiation, the animals were used for the experiment. In Fig.10., growth curves of tumor after irradiation is shown. We observed three kind of growth curve, that is continuously regressed curve, growth stunting curve and later regrown curve. The most prominent influence was observed on the extruding club-like capillaries which were on the surface of the tumor mass. The diameter of these capillaries became thin. Those changes were noticed partially in the

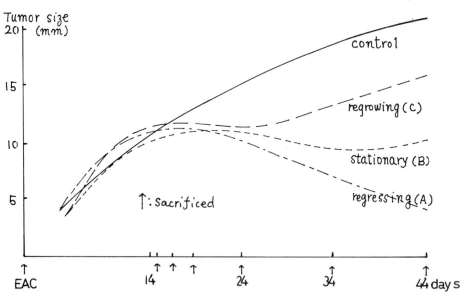

Fig. 10. Growth curve of transplanted tumor, 30 Gy was given at 14 days after transplantation.

tumor (curve A in Fig. 10), through the whole experimental period. The
degree of this change became more prominent later. On the tumor which was
corresponding to curve B, the change was noticed only at 20 days and 30 days
after irradiation. On the tumor which was corresponding to curve C, the
prominent change was not observed at all experimental period. The
thinning of capillary was observed also on the disordered running vessels which
were at the neigbor site of the central necrotic cavity. On the tumor of curve
A, the change could not observe at one and 3 days, but slightly appeared from
5 days, the prominent change could observe at 10, 20 and 30 days after irradiation. But this change was not observed on the tumors of curve B and C at
all experimnetal period (Fig. 11. a, b, c, d.).

In wave-like vessels, tortous vessels, sinusoidal vessels and tapering
vessels, the changes due to irradiation was not observed. The influence of
irradiation on each pattern of capillaries was summarized in Fig. 12.

As a summary, the most affected site of capillary structure was outer layer
of the tumor mass. McAlister, Saeki, Hilmas reported the thiining of capillary
diameter and decrease of blood vessels distribution by irradiation as noticed
by our study.

Patterns of tumor capillary	observation days after irradiation														
	30			20			10			5			3		1	
	A	B	C	A	B	C	A	B	C	A	B	C	A	B	A	B
club-like vessel	╫	+	—	╫	+	—	╫	—	—	╫	—	—	+	—	+	—
disordered vessel	╫	—	—	╫	—	—	╫	—	—	+	—	—	—	—	—	—
tortuous vessel and others	—	—	—	—	—	—	—	—	—	—	—	—	—	—	—	—

A: regressing   B: stationary   C: Regrowing

╫: marked change   +: moderate change   —: no change

Fig. 12 Effect of radiation on the capillary of tumor

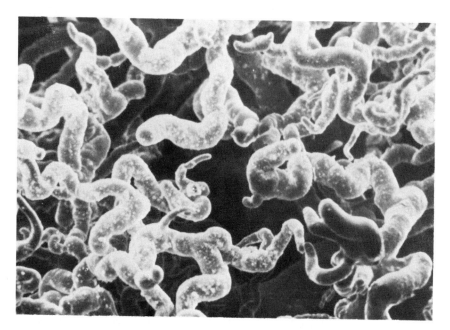

Fig. 11-a. Extruding capillaries on the surface of tumor, no irradiation.

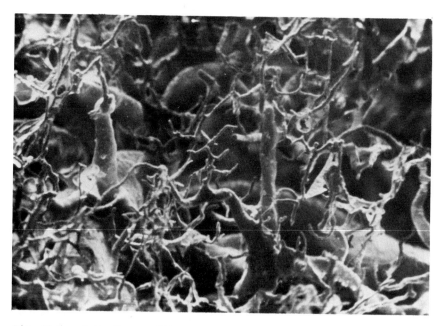

Fig. 11-b. Extruding capillaries, corresponding to curve A in Fig.10.
Thinning and sparse of capillaries are observed. 30 days after irradiation
of 30 Gy.

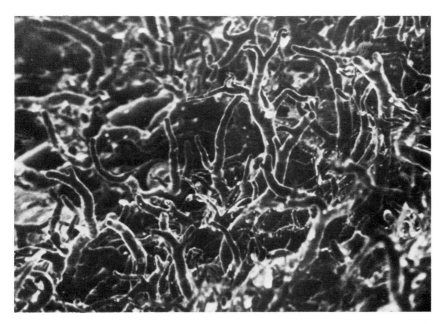

Fig. 11-c. Extruding capillaries of the tumor, 30 days after irradiation of 30 Gy. Corresponding to the curve B.

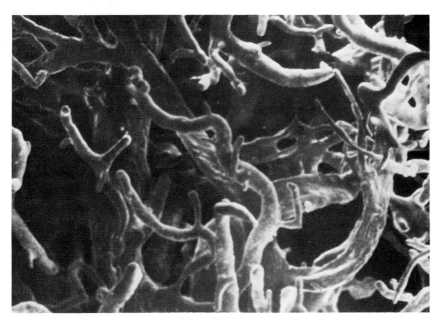

Fig. 11-d. Extruding capillaries of the tumor 30 days after irradiation of 30 Gy. Corresponding to the curve C.

VASCULAR STRUCTURE AND RADIORESISTANCY

The distribution of microvascular system in tumors are closely related to radioresistancy. 1955, Thomlinson and Grey[27] presented a concept of tumor cord. When a cord grew in size, diameter of which is 150 to 200 micron, central necrosis ocurred. Anoxic area of tumors are radioresistant, as shown by many investigators. Rubin and Casarett[15] illustrated the kinetics of progressive central necrosis of an epithelial tumor in three ways. Also they presented the small dose of radiation resulted supervascularization. Second important concept is the reoxygenation. We do not still know the real mechanism of reoxygenation. It may be due to reduced O_2 metabolism, improved circulation, shrinkage of tumors or migration of cell (Kallman[28]). The observation of vascular structure will be useful for the understanding of radioresistance of tumors. Those are the change of capillary construction acording to the tumor growth, the recognition of the site of damage in the vascular structure of tumors and finally measurement of intercapillary distances. By our limited examination and also by the limitation of the method, much cannot be speculated. As the tumor grew, necrotic cavity was formed, here, no vascularizations were observed and the oxygenation may be worsened at the surrounding area of necrosis as observed by the tapering capillaries. By rather large dose (30 Gy) to the tumor, and within the period of observation, outer layer of capillary cast seems to be effected severely, this may correlate to the shrinkage of tumors. The thinning of the disordered vessels were also noticed. The meaning of which is not clarified. The measurement of capillary distance was not possible yet. We have the impression that the capillary network was rather sparse.

SUMMARY

The vascular structure of four kind of experimental tumors was observed by scanning electron microscope using resin cast method. Six patterns of capillary could be identified in the tumor. The appearance and location of the capillary were almost identical in the tumors. The effects of radiation on the capillries were studied. The most prominent changes were observed on the club-like capillary of outer layer and disordered running vessels of inner part of the capillary system. The changes were correlated to the growth patterns of tumors after irradiation.

REFERENCES

1. Angulo, A.W., Hessert, Jr.E.G. and Kownacki, V.P. (1958) Strain Technol., 33, 63-66.

2. Jee, W.S.S. and Arnold, J.S. (1960) Strain Technol., 35, 59-65.

3. Tiboldi, T., Kurcz, M. and Kovács, K. (1968) Neoplasma, 15, 259-265.

4. Margulis, A.R., Carlsson, E. and Mc Alister, W.H. (1961) Acta Radiol., 56, 179-192.

5. Maruyama, K. (1972) J. Japan Surg. Assoc. 73, 1260-1262.

6. Bishton, R.L. and Rogers, G.H. (1950) Nature, 166, 230-231.

7. Rubin, P. Casarett, G.W., et al. (1964) Amer. J. Roentgenol., 92, 378-387.

8. Batson, O,V. (1955) Anat. Rec., 121, 425.

9. Murakami, T. (1971) Arch. Histol. Jap., 32, 445-454.

10. Egawa, J. and Ishioka, K. (1978) Acta Radiol., 17, 414-422.

11. Egawa, J. and Ishioka, K. and Ogata, T. (1979) Acta Radiol. in print.

12. Kawamura, F. and Fujiwara, K. (1973) In: Fraction size in radiobiology and radiotherapy, p. 27.Edited bt T.Sugahara, L.Révész and O.Scott. Igaku Shoin, Tokyo 1973.

13. McAlister, W,H, and Margulis, A.R. (1963) Radiol. 81, 664-674.

14. Saeki, Y., Shimazaki, S. and Urano, M. (1971) Radiology 101, 175-180.

15. Rubin, P. and Casarett, G. (1968) Clinical radiation pathology, Philadelphia, London and Toronto.

16. Kligerman, M.M. and Henel, D.K. (1961) Radiology 76, 810-817.

17. Yamaura, H. and Sato, H. (1974) J.Nat. Cancer Inst., 53, 1229-1240.

18. Hilmas, D.E. and Gillette, E.L. (1975) Radiation Res., 61, 128-243.

19. Reinhold, H.S. and Buisman, G.H. (1973) Brit. J. Radiol., 46, 54-57.

20. Song, C..H. and Levitt, S.H. (1971) Radiology 100, 397-407.

21. Clement, J.J., Tanaka, N. and Song, C.W. (1978) Radiology 127, 799-803.

22. Pochen, E.J. Kinzie, J., Curtis, C. et al. (1972) Cancer. 30, 639-642.

23. Fujiwara, T. (1974) Jap. J. Cancer Clin., 20, 52-54.

24. Tannock, I.F. and Steel, G.G. (1969) J.Nat. Cancer Inst., 42, 771-780.

25. Moss, W.T. and Gold, S. (1963) Amer. Jo Roentgenol., 90, 294-299.

26. Reinhold, H.S. (1971) Europ. J. Cancer 7, 273-280.

27 Thomlinson, R.H. and Gray. L.H. (1955) Brit. J. Cancer 9, 539-549.

28 Kallman, R.F. (1972) Radiology 105, 135-142.

AUTHOR INDEX

230